Yuniel Chávez Mena
Keylan Guzmán Reyes
Yailin Pérez Díaz

Health determinants

Yuniel Chávez Mena
Keylan Guzmán Reyes
Yailin Pérez Díaz

Health determinants

Behavior in type 2 diabetic patients.

ScienciaScripts

Imprint

Any brand names and product names mentioned in this book are subject to trademark, brand or patent protection and are trademarks or registered trademarks of their respective holders. The use of brand names, product names, common names, trade names, product descriptions etc. even without a particular marking in this work is in no way to be construed to mean that such names may be regarded as unrestricted in respect of trademark and brand protection legislation and could thus be used by anyone.

Cover image: www.ingimage.com

This book is a translation from the original published under ISBN 978-3-330-09710-0.

Publisher:
Sciencia Scripts
is a trademark of
Dodo Books Indian Ocean Ltd. and OmniScriptum S.R.L publishing group

120 High Road, East Finchley, London, N2 9ED, United Kingdom
Str. Armeneasca 28/1, office 1, Chisinau MD-2012, Republic of Moldova, Europe
Managing Directors: Ieva Konstantinova, Victoria Ursu
info@omniscriptum.com

Printed at: see last page
ISBN: 978-620-3-56237-8

SUMMARY

Introduction: *One of the diseases on the rise worldwide, caused by the alteration of the social determinants of health is diabetes mellitus.* ***Objective: To*** *describe the behaviour of the social determinants of health associated with type 2 diabetic patients in a clinic in the period from July 2019 to May 2021.* ***Methods:*** *A descriptive, cross-sectional, quantitative-qualitative study was conducted. The population consisted of 59 older adults with type 2 diabetes and the sample was selected by simple random probability sampling, with prior informed consent.* ***Results:*** *Females predominated (54.24%), the age group 75 to 79 years (30.51%), the skin colour was white (88.13%), 30.51% had no schooling, housewives for 37.29%, 64.41% had family history of diabetes, 67.80% had obesity and primary hyperlipoproteinaemias as comorbidity, stress and smoking determinant were found in 100% of subjects, families of diabetics were functional in 61.02%, slight glycaemia uncontrolled (47.45%), as complications neuropathies and heart diseases and high economic status (44.06%).* ***Conclusions:*** *Women aged 75-79 years, white, without schooling, housewives, with a family history of diabetes mellitus, as comorbidities obesity and primary hyperlipoproteinaemias predominated. The social determinants of health that had the greatest impact were stress, smoking, inadequate diet and a predominantly high economic situation.*

Keywords: Social determinants of health, Diabetes mellitus

INDEX

INTRODUCTION

One of the diseases on the rise worldwide, caused by the alteration of the social determinants of health, is diabetes mellitus. This disorder has an endemic character as a result of race, altered lifestyle habits and old age that reach the people who make up a population. [1]

Diabetes mellitus (DM) due to its high morbidity and mortality is among the four major non-communicable diseases that have become one of the greatest development challenges of the 21st century. [2]

The International Diabetes Federation states that type 2 diabetes (T2DM) accounts for the majority of diabetes cases worldwide and has been declared a global health emergency. [3]

Globally, DM affects more than 194 million people and it is estimated that this number will reach 366 million cases by 2030. The growth rate of DM is reported to be higher in developing countries, which can be explained by increasing urbanisation and westernisation of habits and lifestyles. It is among the leading causes of early mortality and disability. [4]

Likewise, the World Health Organisation (WHO) in a report presented in 2020, stated that the overall excess mortality in patients with DM2 is about 15 % higher as of 2020, but varies widely depending on the country. The prevalence of the threatening diabetic disease in the United States is about 4.4 % among adults over the age of 40. [5]

In Mexico City, according to reports presented by the Ministry of Education, Science, Technology and Innovation and the National Institute of Public Health, there are 2.2 million people with DM2 and more than 70% of the inhabitants have predisposing risk factors (overweight or obesity). [6]

Peru has 3-9 cases of diabetes mellitus per 100 inhabitants aged 15 years and older, according to the 2019 Demographic and Family Health Survey (Endes). The previous year (2018), the figure was 0.3% lower in the same segment of residents. [7] Diabetes mellitus is a multisystemic organic syndrome characterised by increased blood glucose levels as a result of defects in insulin secretion. It occurs at any age regardless of sex, race or religion, but adults are the most affected. [8]

Older age, sedentary lifestyle, overweight, family history of diabetes, high blood pressure, impaired glucose tolerance and hyperlipaemia are risk factors that cluster with the increase of the disease. Most cases of type 2 diabetes mellitus originate from a metabolic syndrome in which high blood pressure, increased levels of cholesterol, triglycerides and/or uric acid and obesity are associated.[7]

Studies indicate that most cases of diabetes can be prevented by a healthy diet based on fruits and vegetables and a healthy diet that allows for the maintenance of an adequate body weight, as well as avoiding harmful substances such as tobacco and alcohol, facts and recommendations that in practice are not put into practice due to a lack of health education and fundamentally due to the necessary control by the entities responsible for health administration. [8]

Diabetes mellitus, and chronic non-communicable diseases in general, are pathologies that cannot be effectively addressed without taking into account the social determinants of health. DM, especially type 2, is a disease whose progress is affected by closely related social elements. [1] In recent decades, a field of empirical research has been progressively developing and consolidating with regard to the so-called social determinants of health. health (DSS). This research programme and body of knowledge has confirmed that there are a number of social factors that significantly affect health, leading to different health outcomes between and within populations. [9]

The social determinants of health approach has highlighted the urgent need to look at people's living conditions in order to properly understand the process of health and disease, and thus provide more appropriate responses that improve the health conditions of the population and modify inequalities. [10]

Determining health status is a broad topic that changes from one setting to another, in which determinants interact in a non-linear way. There are determinants that are directly linked to the individual, such as behaviours and habits aimed at caring for health and the usefulness of health-related services. On the other hand, there are those that interact with the social sphere.[1]

Social determinants of health (SDH) provide an opportunity to address DM2 from a broader perspective. SDH is a concept that arises from the need to consider health conditions beyond the human biopsychic nexus in which diseases of great social impact such as DM2 develop. [5]

Diabetes mellitus, specifically type 2 diabetes mellitus, is a condition caused by multiple causes, where social determinants of health, such as income and educational levels, occupation, accessibility to health services, high-calorie diets, physical inactivity, beliefs about beauty, gender and family functioning, are closely related and play a major role, all of which leads to increasing evidence that diabetes mellitus is a social disease. [11]

Type 2 diabetes mellitus is a typical example of a disease that seems to be concentrated in areas of higher poverty and in individuals with low income and low status. educational. This relationship is also conditioned by the role of socio-economic status in health care, disease prevention, health promotion measures, willingness to seek treatment and lifestyles. [12]

In a study on the social determinants of type 2 diabetes mellitus in Ciudad del Este, it was shown that when the various risk factors were linked to the sex variable, 67% of the female population had an inadequate diet and 33% of the male population had an inadequate diet, while a sedentary lifestyle accounted for 67% and 33% of the total cases respectively, Alcoholism affected 8% of the male sex and no cases were detected in the female sex. When exploring the differences in lifestyles of the population studied, significant differences were found in which 50% of the population live in a healthy way, 33% in a moderately healthy way and 17% in an unhealthy way. [13] Authors such as Heredia et al. have investigated DSS and the risk of T2DM in the Mexican population and concluded that the main risk factors for T2DM in the Mexican population are

adults were suffering from high blood pressure while overweight/obesity is a risk factor shared by adults and children. [14]

Rodríguez Plasencia et al., when assessing the social determinants of health in relation to the prevention of diabetic foot disease, determined that 50.0% of the patients have a medium socioeconomic level; 41.3% are of the adult age group; 55.0% are of mixed race; 30.0% have a higher level of education and 21.3% have a temporary and independent employment status.[1]

Marmot classifies social determinants as proximal, intermediate and structural and as conditions that are a product of the political and economic context of each region through which the unequal distribution of goods and services and inequalities can be established. [12]

The American Diabetes Association (ADA) includes recommendations for adapting treatment to the social context, recognising the important role played by the social determinants in diabetes outcomes. For years, the WHO has also been promoting the study of social determinants because they constitute one of the variables for developing a comprehensive and more effective response to health needs. [15]

In Cuba, since 1975, the National Institute of Endocrinology has developed a National Programme of Comprehensive Care for Diabetics, indicating that this disease i s preventable by acting on well-defined risk factors. [16] However, diabetes is one of the ten leading causes of death in the country, occupying eighth place according to national statistics. [17]

According to the Cuban statistical yearbook, in 2019, DM had a prevalence of 66.7 per 1000 inhabitants and Villa Clara province 66.9, ranking seventh at the national level. Therefore, it is necessary to study type 2 diabetes in adults, given that a high number of patients in the municipality are affected. In addition, in the South Polyclinic there is a high increase in the prevalence of this disease in the 2019 dispensary, with 1989 cases and an incidence of 96 patients, equivalent to 4.82%, reporting 45 more diabetics than in 2018 and the fact that the 14-32 clinic has 77 type 2 diabetics, where 76.6% are aged 60 years and over, based on a constricted population pyramid with a tendency to be stationary. In addition, it is known that these patients frequently come for consultation due to uncontrolled glycaemia, complications and admissions associated with deterioration in quality of life and complications as the main causes of morbidity and mortality, so it was decided to pose this as a research problem:

Scientific problem: What is the behaviour of the health determinants associated with type 2 diabetic patients in the 14-32 clinic of the Placetas South Polyclinic in the period from July 2019 to May 2021?

OBJECTIVES

General objective: To describe the behaviour of the social determinants of health associated with type 2 diabetic patients in the 14-32 clinic in Área Sur in the period from July 2019 to May 2021.

Specific objectives:

1. Characterise the sample according to clinical and epidemiological variables of interest in the research.

2. To identify the social determinants of health that most affect the patients studied.

3. To establish associations between the social determinants investigated, glycaemic control and the complications detected.

THEORETICAL FRAMEWORK

Non-communicable diseases are a public health problem that generates a large amount o f financial resources d u e to the high costs of care required for their management. [18]

Chronic non-communicable diseases (NCDs) such as DM2 are complex and represent a global challenge for society and health systems. The global prevalence of DM2 has been attributed to a complex set of socioeconomic, demographic and environmental factors and an increase in risk factors for developing the disease related to unhealthy lifestyles, such as overweight/obesity and low levels of physical activity. [5, 14]

History

Diabetes is a disease that has been known since ancient times, the first written reference to which we have evidence is from ancient Egypt, around 1553 BC. Near Luxor, the archaeologist George Ebers found a papyrus that refers to diabetes and describes one of its main symptoms, polyuria, an increase in urine production. [19]

In the 5th or 3rd century BC, the Indian physician Susruta described a strange disease, typical of rich, obese people who ate a lot of sweets and rice and whose characteristic was a sticky urine, with a sweet taste and which attracted ants and flies, which is why they called it madhumeha (honey urine). In this way Susruta, the father of Hindu medicine, described diabetes mellitus, calling it the "disease of the rich", e v e n classifying it into a diabetes that occurred in the young that led to death and another that occurred in people of a certain age. He also explains that this disease usually affected several members of the same family. The term diabetes from the Greek "that which goes through" was first used by Aretaeus of Cappadocia (81-133 A.D.) in his treatise "On the Causes and Symptoms of diseases" also describes excessive thirst and increased urination (polydipsia).

and polyuria), with increased appetite (polyphagia) going unnoticed at this time. In the 2nd century Galen considered diabetes to be a kidney disease, and that it was the abundant urine that caused cachexia because the body was unable to retain the liquid. Persia Avicenna (980-1037) writes about diabetes in his book "Canon de la

Medicine", identifying increased appetite, problems with the sexual system, the gangrene and the sweetness of urine. Later, Paracelsus (1493-1541) considered that diabetes was not a kidney disease as was commonly accepted until then, but a blood disease. He boiled the urine of a patient and obtained white crystals which, without testing them, he considered to be salt, which according to him explained the abundant sensation of thirst and urine of diabetics.

Thomas Willis coined the term mellitus in 1672 when he discovered that the urine of these patients was sweet. This served to establish a diagnostic difference from other causes of polyuria.

Claude Bernard (1813-1878) investigated how certain foods can be converted into glucose (1857), and how the liver converts glycogen, which can then be converted back into glucose, to maintain constant plasma levels. His research described two diagnostic criteria f o r diabetes mellitus: hyperglycaemia and glycosuria.

In 1919 Frederick Allen (1879-1964) proposed the treatment of diabetes through a diet very low in carbohydrates. In 1921 Frederick G. Bantin and Charles H. Best had the idea of

7

ligating the pancreatic excretory duct of a monkey, causing the gland to self-digest. Then, by squeezing out what was left of this pancreas, they obtained a liquid that managed to lower blood glucose levels: this is how insulin was discovered. The first injection of insulin in humans was given to a 14-year-old boy named Leonard Thompson on 11 December January 1922 at the Toronto Hospital in Canada.[19] In terms of technological developments in diabetes management, the first insulin pens appeared in 1985. From 1980 onwards, the manufacture of human recombinant insulins marked a major breakthrough in the treatment of diabetes. diabetes. Richard K. Bernstein developed the first portable glucometer. [20]

In the field of artificial pancreas it led to the appearance of the first commercial system in June 2017: the Medtronic minimed™ 670G system. [21]

Epidemiology

The World Health Organisation (WHO), in 2019, stated that diabetes was the sixth leading cause of death with an estimated 244,084 people dying as a result of complications, including kidney failure, cardiac arrest, stroke and loss of lower limbs.[1]

According to the International Diabetes Federation (IDF), approximately 415 million adults between the ages of 40 and 79 have diabetes mellitus and this number is expected to increase to 693 million by 2045. [5]

Approximately 62 million people in the Americas have diabetes. Most live in low- and middle-income countries, and 244,084 deaths are directly attributed to diabetes annually. The number of cases of type II diabetes is steadily increasing over the past decades. [7]

The countries with the largest number of people with diabetes are China, which has more than 116 million people with diabetes. In second place is India with more than 77 million. In third place is the United States with around 31 million. [22]

In the United States, an estimated 30.3 million individuals suffer from diabetes, representing 9.4% of the total population, of which 12 million people are aged 65 years or older; North America and the Caribbean account for 11%, the Middle East and North Africa 10.8%, Southeast Asia 10.1%, Europe 6.8% and in the United States 6.8%. prevalence of diabetes mellitus in the western world is 20%.[23] By 2030, 11.2% of US adults are expected to have the condition. [5]

In Mexico the picture is no different, according to official data from 2018 the prevalence of T2DM in 2018 was 10.3% and it is the third leading cause of death in the country. [14]

Two of the top ten countries with the highest number of cases are in Latin America: Brazil with 14.3 million and Mexico with 11.5 million cases, respectively. [6] According to the WHO (2018), there are approximately 2 million people in Peru who suffer from diabetes and it is the fifteenth leading cause of death. The same organisation predicts that deaths from diabetes will double between 2005 and 2030. Mortality from diabetes in people between 30 and 69 years of age in men was 710 and in women 640; and in those aged 70 and over, in men it was 750 and in women 850. [8]

In Ecuador, 7.8% of Ecuadorians have high blood glucose levels, and according to data obtained by the Ministry of Public Health, diabetes has been responsible for 34,597 diagnoses, only up to half of the year 2018, where only 1.82% of the cases are type 1 diabetes mellitus. In the years between 2014 and 2017, according to INEC, diabetes is the second leading cause of death. [24] The prevalence of the disease in Uruguay is 8.2% of the adult population, according to official data. [25]

According to the American Diabetes Association (ADA), Diabetes Mellitus is defined as a set of metabolic disorders characterised by chronic hyperglycaemia, which is the result of a failure in insulin secretion, in the effects of insulin, or both. It is classified into 4 groups:

• Type 1 Diabetes Mellitus: characterised by autoimmune destruction of pancreatic Beta cells. Type 2 diabetes mellitus: the defect consists of insulin resistance accompanied by insulin deficiency.

• Gestational diabetes: a rise in glucose for the first time in pregnancy.

• Other specific types of diabetes: this group includes a wide variety of rare conditions. [6, 26]

Diabetes Mellitus type 2

Concept

Arpita Laruta et al. state that type 2 diabetes mellitus is a chronic, multifactorial disease, distinguished by a carbohydrate metabolic disorder, deficient in insulin secretion or action, leading to chronic hyperglycaemia causing microvascular and macrovascular complications. [7] Type 2 diabetes is generally defined as hyperglycaemia resulting from an imbalance between insulin production and the body's adequate response to it. It has always been a disease that primarily affects adults while type 1 diabetes is associated with paediatric ages, although this is not always the case. [27]

Limón García et. al. state that TD2 is defined as the inability of the body's cells to respond fully to insulin and is influenced by various factors, traditionally non-modifiable (age, female sex,2 hereditary family history 1 of first line) and modifiable (weight, high-calorie diets, high body mass index, total cholesterol, obesity, hyperglycaemia, inadequate diet,3 high waist circumference, HTN, sedentary lifestyle and socioeconomic status). [3] The author is affiliated with the concept put forward by Limón García et. al. as she considers it to be the one that most comprehensively sets out the characteristics and risk factors of the pathology.

Risk factors for Diabetes Mellitus type 2

DM2 is a disease caused by a combination of genetic, environmental and behavioural factors. The predisposing risk factors can be divided into:

• Modifiable risk factors: obesity, overweight, abdominal obesity, sedentary lifestyle, smoking and dietary patterns,

• Non-modifiable risk factors: age, race, history of DM2 in a first-degree relative, history of gestational DM, polycystic ovary syndrome. [6, 28]

Pathophysiology

Hepatic and muscular insulin resistance are attributed the main responsibility for the aetiopathogenesis of DM-2. Increased hepatic glucose synthesis and decreased glucose uptake by muscle would lead to a progressive increase in blood glucose levels, which, together with deficient insulin secretion by the pancreatic beta-cell, would determine the onset of the clinical picture of DM-2.

The involvement of other components in the progression of DM-2 such as adipose tissue, gastrointestinal tissue, pancreatic islet alpha cell, kidney and brain has now been demonstrated. [29]

Clinical manifestations

It can produce signs and symptoms such as: [30]

❑ Abnormal thirst and dry mouth❑ Extreme hunger
❑ Frequent urination❑ Lack of energy
❑ Extreme tiredness

❑ Sudden weight loss

❑ Slow healing wounds❑ Recurrent infections
❑ Blurred vision Pathophysiology

In the early years, a long preclinical period of insulin resistance predominates, in which the pancreas progressively increases insulin secretion to compensate for this alteration, producing hyperinsulinaemia, which maintains normal fasting and postprandial blood glucose levels, and is also associated with lipotoxicity in patients with obesity and insulin resistance. In a second stage, there is an acute response in which the insulin resistance response is maintained, but the secretory capacity of the B cells begins to decrease, increasing blood glucose levels and manifesting itself in the laboratory finding of altered fasting blood glucose levels and glucose intolerance figures. [31]

Clinical complications of type II diabetes

Complications from diabetes account for 91% of lower limb amputations, 60% of hospitalisations due to cardiovascular disease and 50% of hospitalisations due to stroke. Approximately a quarter of diabetes deaths are due to complications of the disease. [15]

Complications that can arise as a result of type II diabetes can be acute and chronic or long-term. [5]

Acute complications are hyperglycaemia, hypoglycaemia and diabetic ketoacidosis. Long-term or chronic complications increase in severity depending on the level of glucose control the person has maintained throughout their disease. In the long term, the most common are retinopathy, nephropathy, neuropathy and cardiovascular disease. Similarly, amputations, dental disease, pregnancy complications and sexual dysfunction are associated with a diagnosis of diabetes. [5,32] Chronic complications of diabetes mellitus include:

0 Ophthalmological: non-proliferative or proliferative diabetic retinopathy, macular oedema, iris rubeosis, glaucoma and cataracts.

0 Renal: proteinuria, end-stage renal disease and type IV renal tubular acidosis.

0 Neurological: distal symmetrical polyneuropathy, polyradiculopathy, mononeuropathy and autonomic neuropathy.

0 Gastrointestinal: gastroparesis, diarrhoea and constipation.

O Genitourinary: cystopathy, erectile dysfunction, sexual dysfunction in women and vaginal candidiasis.

O Cardiovascular: coronary artery disease, congestive heart failure, peripheral vascular disease and stroke. Lower extremities: foot deformity (hammer toe, claw toe and Charcot foot), ulcers and amputation.

O Dermatological: infections (folliculitis, furunculosis, cellulitis), necrobiosis, poor healing, ulcers and gangrene. Dental: periodontal disease. [7]

Prevention

Prevention of DM2 is divided into three main levels:

• Primary: aims to prevent the onset of the disease in two age groups: the general population (lifestyle modifiers and socio-environmental characteristics) and the population with risk factors associated with diabetes (health education, correction of obesity, appropriate prescription of medication, promotion of routine and programmed exercise).

• Secondary: for those with an established diagnosis of DM2, the goals will be to prevent, avoid or delay acute complications.

• Tertiary: aimed at patients who already have chronic complications and aims to prevent disability from kidney failure, blindness, diabetic foot and early death. [6]

Social determinants of health

Background

Social determinants of health (SDH) have been considered for more than 100 years, where Rudolph Virchow, the prominent 19th century German pathologist and other contemporaries of his, referred to living conditions as determinants of the health conditions of the population. Virchow referred that "medicine is a social science and politics is nothing but medicine on a broader scale". [10]

In 1948, Flenry Singer argued that health would be provided to people when decent living and working conditions were promoted), so he proposed that the government should carry out what he called "health promotion". [33]

The DSS were addressed by Mare Lalonde in 1974, who, from an epidemiological point of view, discusses the major causes of death and disease in Canadians. [33]

The concept of DSS originated as a result of a series of critical analyses that were published in the 1970s and 1980s. [10] The WHO launched the Commission on Social Determinants of Health in 2005, which called for a model to address the underlying social, economic and political causes of ill-health. [10, 33, 34]

In October 2011, the World Conference on Social Determinants of Health was held in Rio de Janeiro, which adopted a declaration that was subsequently adopted by the 65th World Health Assembly in May 2012. [9]

HSSD, according to WHO, are understood as "... the circumstances in which people are born, grow, live, work and age, including the health system. [10,33,35-37] These circumstances are the result of global, national and local circumstances, which in turn depend on the policies adopted. [10,33,38]

Another definition is that proposed by Tarlov, in which he conceives of SDH as "the social characteristics within which life takes place". They have a significant and vital influence on the improvement of the health of individuals. [34] These factors are found in different proportions in each region or country, depending on the socio-political, economic and cultural circumstances of each. [35]

The author agrees with the concept given by the World Health Organisation, which encompasses all social, economic and geographical aspects, making it comprehensible without losing academic rigour.

Current situation

In short, research on the social determinants of health has been systematically linking social conditions of advantage and disadvantage to health outcomes. For example, in the UK, where there is a National Health Service with universal coverage, the difference in life expectancy of professionals and managers compared to manual workers is almost 10 years. The latter is probably one of the most striking aspects of the research on the social determinants of health: social position has an enormous relevance for health outcomes, even independently of access to health care. To this must be added another striking finding of this research, namely that these health differences do not only occur at the extremes, but also along the social scale, in what is known as the socio-economic gradient. [9]

In Latin America, structural reforms have been carried out in the constitutions of several countries that seek to adjust health systems to a PHC model; at the same time, there have been implemented public health policies to intervene on SHR from various spheres. For example, in Argentina, there are public policies aimed at improving the health of indigenous populations by improving intercultural dialogue, which facilitates social participation and makes health care more inclusive. 39 In Mexico, the Ministry of Health was in charge of giving its health plan a DSS approach, which led to the creation of programmes to combat extreme poverty, with an emphasis on women and vulnerable populations. The case of Chile is different, with the creation of a technical secretariat for SHD that promoted strategies to influence the determinants affecting the most vulnerable populations. In Colombia, the ten-year public health plan was implemented with a DSS approach that sought to address inequalities in various areas. 39 On the other hand, although countries such as Cuba have included the teaching of SHD in their undergraduate medical training, PHC plays a fundamental role in the successful inclusion of these pedagogical alternatives insofar as it can generate spaces in which clinical care is articulated with SHD. PHC plays a fundamental role in the successful inclusion of these pedagogical alternatives to the extent that it can generate spaces in which clinical care is articulated with DSS. To this end, several models have been created, such as community-oriented primary care, which seeks to give the community an active role in conjunction with health professionals, in order to efficiently distribute available health resources and promote healthy lifestyles. [39]

Within these determinants, the WHO identifies factors such as the unequal distribution of power, income and goods and services, access to health care, schooling and education, working conditions, and the state of housing and the physical environment. [37]

Models of Social Determinants At the second meeting of the Commission on Social Determinants of Health, the models proposed by the following were considered as influential:[36]

O Dahlgren and Whitehead: Layered influences, explains how social inequalities in health are the result of interactions between different levels of causal conditions, from the individual to communities to the level of national health policies.

O Diderichsen et al: Social stratification and the disease of production, This model emphasises how social contexts create social stratification and assign individuals to different social positions, which determines their health status.

According to Adolfo et al., the social production of health and, therefore, its determination, is a result of the social system in place, the prevailing ideology and the dominant culture, so that each country has a very particular characterisation of its own determinants, some common to many and others very particular to each case.

O Among the classical models, the holistic model of Laframbroise (1973), developed by Marc Lalonde (1974), Canadian Minister of Health, in the document New Perspectives on the Health of Canadians, is particularly relevant. According to Lalonde, the level of health of a community would be influenced by four major groups:36

1. Lifestyles and health behaviours: When a lifestyle becomes detrimental to our health, it is a risk factor. Unhealthy diets; physical inactivity; tobacco, alcohol and other drug use; psycho-social stress; and other risky behaviours, such as unprotected sex or reckless driving, are some of the risk factors.

2. Human biology: This includes all those that depend on the biological structure and constitution of the human organism, such as the following:

❑ Genetics. Human beings receive a genetic inheritance that conditions their constitution and the appearance of certain diseases.

❑ Age. The disease tends to be more prevalent in old age because the body does not respond in the same way to stressors.

❑ Gender. Many diseases have a different distribution according to the sex of the patient.

3. Environment: These include the following:

❑ Physical factors: noise pollution, temperature variations, radiation, quality of drinking water and sewage systems, among others.

❑ Chemical factors: e.g. chemical pollution caused by, among others, carbon dioxide, heavy metals, insecticides or pollution.

❑ Biological factors: the micro-organisms that can affect our health are highly variable, such as bacteria, viruses, fungi and parasites.

❑ Psychological and socio-cultural factors: relationships with family and friends, working conditions, leisure time, unemployment, aggressiveness and violence, degree of stress, etc.

4. Health care system: poor use of resources, adverse health care events, excessive waiting

lists, bureaucratisation of care
Ranking

In keeping with their instrumental sense, the dimensions of the SDGs can be broken down into indicators at the micro, regional and macro levels:

At the micro level, there is a need for social cohesion processes, where supportive social networks reinforce social loyalty, as a positive function of physical and mental health.

Intermediate determinants comprise the various biological and behavioural factors, socio-environmental and psychosocial circumstances, as well as material circumstances (where access to health services would be a key issue).

At the macro level would be the socio-economic and political contexts, i.e. governance, macroeconomic policies, social and public policies, as well as cultural and social values'. [33]

Robles et al. state that the basic components of the conceptual framework of the social determinants of health include: a) the socio-economic and political context; b) the social and political context; c) the social and political context; and d) the social and political context.

b)   structural determinants.

c)   intermediary determinants. [34]

Heredia et al. argue that DSS are composed of structural and intermediate determinants. [14]

Structural determinants comprise the political and socio-economic context (governance, macroeconomic policies, public policies, social policies, culture and social values) and socio-economic position (social class, gender, race, income, occupation, education). [40]

Intermediate determinants include material circumstances (housing quality, consumption potential, working conditions), psychosocial factors (stress, social support) and behaviours (healthy behaviours) and biological factors. [40]

The complexity of the causal connections between broader determinants and health is intricate. But in a general way it can be said that social injustices are ultimately embedded in individuals in the form of disease or, as Farmer puts it, social, political and economic forces are embodied (embody) in individual experiences and structure the risk of disease. [9]

Socially determined processes do not act like biological, physical or chemical agents in the generation of disease, they have no aetiological specificity, nor do they obey a dose-response mechanics. [10]

As health is anchored to the position in the social structure v welfare, government intervention is necessary to generate adequate conditions for the health of the population. population through public policies: that is, the presence of some kind of social state or welfare state is necessary. [33]

Medical care can prolong survival by resolving the circumstances caused by illness. However, the social and economic conditions that determine whether or not people get sick are more important for the health gains of the population as a whole, i.e. conditions of poverty lead to poorer health. [10]

Social determinants of health and type 2 diabetes mellitus Structural determinants

❖   ☐ Socio-economic factor

Health inequalities by socio-economic status tend to increase because people from more advantaged social classes improve their health more than the rest of the population. [18] People of lower socio-economic status may face a sense of subordination and lack of control that can lead to chronic stress and deteriorating health. [32] Education level influences employment opportunities, self-care and general health. [31]

Communicable diseases such as acute respiratory infections, gastrointestinal infections, intestinal amebiasis, conjunctivitis and others are related to indicators of poverty (limited access to drinking water and drainage, dirt floors, and limited access to health care).

acquisitive). [41] ❖ Sex:

There is little gender difference in the global number of people with diabetes from 2015 to 2040. There are about 15.6 million more men than women with diabetes 215.2 million men vs. 199.5 million women. [18] Guerra et. al. state that a higher frequency of type 2 diabetes mellitus has been observed in women, which is linked to cultural aspects and low income as a consequence of the social disadvantages to which women are still exposed in many regions of the world. [30] Racial or ethnic groups:

Certain genes can make a person more prone to type II diabetes. The disease has a hereditary tendency and occurs more often in these racial or ethnic groups: [18,42]

• African Americans

• Alaska Natives

• American Indians

• Asian Americans

• Hispanic or Latino

• Native Hawaiians

• Pacific Islander ❖□ Education:

Prevalence varied significantly by educational attainment, which is an indicator of socioeconomic status. Specifically, 12.6 % of adults with less than an upper secondary school education had diagnosed diabetes, compared to 9.5 % of those with an upper secondary school education and 9.5 % of those with an upper secondary school education.

7.2 % of those who had reached a higher level. [18] ❖ Occupation: is the individual's position within the social structure, which helps to protect them from certain occupational hazards, facilitates their access to health resources, produces different levels of psychological stress and can influence their behaviour or the adoption of healthy lifestyles. [30]

Intermediate determinants ❖ Age:

It refers to the fact that the older you are, the more likely you are to develop pre-diabetes or type 2 diabetes, as this condition occurs mostly in adults. [28]

❖ Stress and well-being:

Many people experience stress, but not everyone reacts in the same way, therefore, it is important to manage stress in our lives, as it allows us to have a good control of a healthy lifestyle. [28]

When a person feels tense too often, or when that tension is sustained for too long, he or she becomes more vulnerable to a wide range of conditions including infections, diabetes, high blood pressure, and other health problems. high blood pressure, heart attacks, strokes, depression and aggression. [30] Weight: The presence of obesity and overweight increases the risk of developing diabetes.28

'Û Alcohol:

Consuming too much alcohol causes inflammation in the pancreas, thereby limiting its ability to produce the hormone insulin.28, 32

'Û Physical inactivity.

Sedentary lifestyles, in both adults and children, are a risk factor for developing type II diabetes. The less physical activity, the greater the risk of developing diabetes as it helps to control weight, uses glucose for energy and makes cells more sensitive to insulin. [30, 42,43]

'Û Inadequate nutrition.

In principle, the negative effects of poor nutrition are a clear reflection of today's hectic lifestyle, which leaves many people with insufficient time to prepare and consume healthy food and meals.

The most common unhealthy foods include highly processed foods. "Just like fast food and snack foods," highly processed foods tend to be low in nutrients (vitamins, minerals and antioxidants) and high in empty calories because they contain refined flour, sodium and sugar.[42]

Similarly, in poor or low-income strata, these conditions are observed in addition to malnutrition associated with poor diets, characterised by an excess of foods rich in fats (especially saturated fats), refined and simple sugars and poor in complex carbohydrates (fibre), an increase in industrialised, low-cost, energy-dense and poor quality foods and drinks, which have been replacing the traditional diet30 , without taking into account the affectation among the population. children and adolescents. This dietary pattern contributes to the presence of DM. [44]

Obesity

It is considered to be the basis for the possible development of diabetes mellitus due to the metabolic disorder that the body starts to suffer from. Obese individuals already begin to suffer from hyper-insulinaemia due to the constant stress on the pancreas as it releases the hormone. In relation to this, Rubin says that obesity increases people's resistance to their own insulin through a hormone secreted by fat cells called "resistin", which causes insulin resistance. [31]

Smoking

It is a strong cardiovascular risk factor that is not included in the definition of metabolic syndrome (MS) but substantially increases the risk of microvascular and macrovascular complications in patients with type 2 DM (DM2), while smoking cessation substantially reduces this risk. Given that exposure to cigarette smoke is associated with vascular damage, endothelial dysfunction and activation of coagulation and fibrinolysis, it is not surprising that smoking increases the combined deleterious effects of elevated blood glucose and other risk factors and accelerates vascular damage.

in patients with diabetes. [45] ❖ Family functioning

In this sense, in general, living with a partner has been shown to be associated with a better health profile compared to the non-partnered counterpart population. This difference has been justified by the optimisation of resources through economies of scale within the partner context, or by the creation and maintenance of a larger social network that can be of help in the face of possible disadvantages. [46]

Diabetes Mellitus has claimed lives due to poor lifestyles and contributing factors such as poor diet, obesity, the use of psychotropic drugs, family neglect, which results from family dysfunction.47

The management of type II diabetes involves behavioural change, which is achieved through family intervention. You can change your eating habits together. This will reduce the amount of unhealthy food you have in the house and reduce the feeling of isolation. [48]

The fact that Diabetes Mellitus type 2 is one of the most prevalent chronic diseases, the need to control it properly in order to delay the occurrence of complications and the consequent deterioration in quality of life, and the need to understand the social determinants in order to investigate how these can affect the health of individuals in one way or another, especially those who are less favoured, stimulated the development of the present study.

METHODOLOGY TYPE OF STUDY

A quantitative-qualitative, descriptive and cross-sectional study was carried out with the aim of describing the behaviour of health determinants associated with type 2 diabetic patients in a clinic in the period July 2019 to May 2021.

Population and Sample

The population consisted of 59 type 2 diabetics aged 60 years and over at the clinic. **The sample** was selected probabilistically, through simple random sampling, by way of lottery, of 50, equivalent to 84.7% of the population, with the willingness and approval of the informed consent request of each case resident in the health area. (Annex 1) **Empirical methods**:

• **Documentary analysis**: The analysis of the Family Doctor Programme and the National Programme for Comprehensive Care of Diabetics was carried out. Family records and individual clinical histories were also reviewed to select and characterise the study sample (Annex 2).

• **Semi-structured individual questionnaire**: designed to identify personal data and opinions (Annex 3).

• **Stress Vulnerability Scale Test.** This is an adaptation of the Self-Analysis Model of Le. H. Miller and Smith with the aim of identifying this problem in patients as a very important determinant associated with diabetes (Appendix 4).

• **Family Functioning Test (FF-SIL)** to assess the type of family according to its functioning (Annex 5).

• **Data triangulation**. Qualitative technique to establish regularities, strengths and weaknesses.

Statistical-mathematical methods: Descriptive analysis was carried out according to the level of measurement of the variables using descriptive statistics: frequency tables. expressed in absolute numbers and percentages, t h e rate, mode, mean, median, proportion and ratio. The chi-square test was used for inferential statistics.

Definition and operationalisation of variables.

-Sex: Nominal qualitative. According to biological condition. Scale of measurement:

Female Male

-Age. Discrete quantitative. Expressed in years from birth to the time of t h e research. Scale of measurement.

• 60 to 64 years

• 65 a 69

• 70 a 74

• 75 a 79

• 80 and over

-Skin colour: Qualitative nominal. According to skin colour. Scale of measurement: White Non-white (includes black and mixed race)

-Level of schooling: Qualitative ordinal. According to level of education attained. Scale of measurement.
• Out of school

• Primary

• Secondary

• Skilled worker

• Medium technician

• Pre-university

• University

-Occupation. Nominal qualitative. According to the main activity or occupation carried out at t h e time of the research. Scale of measurement.
• State worker

• Self-employed

• Retired

• Housewife

• Carer of another elderly person or sick relative

• Patient being cared for by a relative or other person

-History of diabetic family members. Nominal qualitative. According to the presence of diabetic first-line relatives: mother, father, grandparents and siblings. [49] Scale of measurement.
  No previous history

 With antecedents. Specify which ones: mother, father, grandparents and siblings - **Associated comorbidity:** Qualitative nominal. According to the presence of other diseases associated with diabetes or concomitant with it,[49] considering the clinical history, as well as the interview. Measurement scale.
Arterial hypertension. All patients with a definitive diagnosis of the disease, with figures above 140/90, were taken into account. [50] Measurement scale YesNo

Obesity. A marked increase in body weight was considered, calculated by the body mass index (BMI)[49] as follows: BMI $= $ Weight (kg)/Height (m^2) where the ranges are:
Low weight: < 18.5 Kg/m^2

Normal: 18.5 Kg/m^2 - 24.9 Kg/m^2

Overweight: 25 - 29.9 Kg/m^2

Obese: ☐ 30 kg/m^2 Scale of measurement Yes No

Primary Hyperlipoproteinaemia: An increase in serum cholesterol level above (5.2mmol/l) and triglycerides (TGC): above (1.8mmol/l) was considered high risk:[49] Yes No

History of Ischaemic Heart Disease. Patients were considered to have suffered episodes of Angina Pectoris (precordial pain with or without electrocardiographic changes, or of a previous AMI)[51] Measuring scale YesNo

Chronic kidney disease. Any diagnosis that directly points to it or the presence of symptoms and signs of its manifestation in early stages of the disease was considered. [32]Scale of measurement.   Yes No

Others, which ones

-Complications: Qualitative nominal. The sequelae of uncontrolled blood glucose, whether acute or chronic, were considered. [51] Measurement scale.

Diabetic foot ulcer. Yes No

Diabetic retinopathy. Yes No

Diabetic neuropathy Yes No

Nephropathy. Yes No

Heart disease Yes No

Other, mention which one.

-Lifestyle determinants:

• **Smoking**. This refers to the use of tobacco or its derivatives. The WHO criteria were considered. (2016). [52] Scale of measurement:

Light smoker: less than 5 cigarettes per day. Moderate smoker: 6 to 15 cigarettes per day. Severe smoker: more than 16 cigarettes per day.

Ex-smoker: when the patient so refers, regardless of the time elapsed.

• **Alcoholism**. When you consume more than one glass of wine (300 mL) daily or exceed the 60 mL limit for whiskey (rum) or the 650 mL limit for beer and beer derivatives. [50]   Yes N o

• **Sedentary lifestyle**. Absence reported by the individual of regularly planned physical activity, as a function of body weight control. [49] The following were considered: Yes No

• **Inadequate diet**: This was considered when the patient's diet is high in saturated fat, i.e. when the patient consumes more than 30 % saturated fat (butter) in the diet, if the sodium intake is more than 5 g per day, which is equivalent to one level teaspoon of salt per capita/day or more than 50-60 % simple carbohydrates (sugar, honey, molasses, soft drinks) [0]– Yes No

• **Stress:** This was considered if you accumulated 24 points or more when answering the questionnaire: Stress Vulnerability Scale (Annex 4) Yes No

• **Family functioning**. Qualitative ordinal. According to the results of the application of the Test to evaluate Family Functioning. FF-SIL (annex 5) Measurement scale:

1- Cohesion: physical and emotional family togetherness in coping with different situations and in decision-making in daily tasks (items 1 and 8).

2- Harmony: matching individual interests and needs with those of the family in a positive emotional balance (items 2 and 13).

3- Communication: family members are able to convey their experiences and knowledge clearly and directly (Items 5 and 11).

4-Adaptability: abilityof the family to change its power structure, role relationships and rules in a situation that requires it (items 6 and 10).

5-Affectivity: ability of family members to experience and demonstrate positive feelings and emotions to each other (items 4 and 14).

6-Role: each family member fulfils the responsibilities and functions negotiated by the household (items 3 and 9).

7-Permeability: the family's ability to provide and receive experiences from other families and institutions (items 7 and 12).

70 to 57 points. Functional family

56 to 43 points. Moderately functional family 42 to 28 points. Dysfunctional Family

27 to 14 points:Severely dysfunctional family

- **Glycaemic control.** Qualitative ordinal. According to the control criteria of the bedside text in the training of General Practitioners in Cuba by Álvarez Sintes et.al.,[50] since it is assumed that good metabolic control is the most effective measure known to avoid or postpone complications. Patients were categorised as follows: Measurement scale:

✓ **Well controlled:**

a) No clinical symptoms of hyperglycaemia.

b) Fasting and postprandial venous plasma glucose less than 140 mg/dL (7.8 mmol/L) 80% of the time when tested.

c) Analyses performed: aglucosurics for 24 h and cholesterol less than 240 mg/dL (6.2 mmol/L).

✓ **Slight decontrol**

a) No symptoms of hyperglycaemia.

b) Fasting or postprandial blood glucose less than 180 mg/dL (10 mmol/L) in venous plasma, 80% of the time when tested.

c) 24 h glycosuria less than 5% of ingested carbohydrate 80% o f   partial glycosuria negative.

d) Cholesterol less than 240 mg/dL (6.2 mmol/L ✓)

Serious lack of control.

Includes the rest of the cases: if the diabetic's glycaemic metabolic control is not adequately achieved with oral hypoglycaemic agents and there are no explanatory factors such as infections, dietary transgressions, psychological disorders, etc., an interconsultation will be made to assess the initiation of insulin treatment.

-Economic situation: Qualitative ordinal. The average economic income of the family was taken into account, according to the current Social Security standard. Qualitative ordinal variable. Measuring scale: o High: more than 5060 pesos o Medium High: 3810 to 5060 pesos o Medium: between 2100 and 3809 pesos
o Medium Low: From 1528 to 2099 pesos (minimum wage of the country) o Low: Less than the minimum pension 1528 pesos

Information processing:

Statistical processing was performed on an Intel computer using Microsoft Excel 2016 for Windows. The quantitative data collected were organised in contingency tables and figures to summarise and present the information in absolute and relative frequencies such as: per cent, rate, mode, mean, ratio and proportion. Also, from the inferential statistics, hypothesis testing was applied to compare percentages based on the probability distribution named Chi-square to identify significant differences between categories and to assess the possible association between qualitative variables. A 95% confidence interval was set. It was used as the level of significance: $p<0.01$ highly significant differences $p<0.01$ and > 0.05 significant differences $p<0.01$ and > 0.05 significant differences $p < 0.05$ no significant difference The qualitative results were summarised in boxes.

Procedures:

A review of the patients' Family Health Histories was carried out to identify those patients with type 2 diabetes, who were selected by means of a random draw. In addition, individual records were reviewed to characterise the study sample and collect information on the variables of interest to the study (Annex 2. Documentary Review Guide).
Subsequently, these patients were visited in their homes, the objectives of the research were explained to them and their request for informed consent was collected, guaranteeing their anonymity by means of a number assigned to each one. In this way, the sample was formed, previously leaving the appointment: day and time, in the afternoon, for the individual interview and the application of the proposed tests: Stress Vulnerability Scale and the FF-SIL. However, if the conditions allowed it, the interview was carried out at that time; nevertheless, it is in the author's interest to plan these interviews and to plan them in advance as part of the follow-up of these patients.
The questionnaire was administered at home, in privacy, taking into account the age of the patients and the fact that they may have some associated health problems and disabilities. In such cases, the doctor, without suggesting the answers, explained what the questionnaire was about, always achieving good doctor-patient communication and the latter giving logical and

coherent answers. When the patient showed signs or symptoms of mental disability to answer about their health-illness status, they were withdrawn from the study because the data obtained were not reliable and to avoid bias in the research. The entire research process was carried out in the area occupied by clinic 1432 in the municipality of Placetas, in the afternoon and field work for the follow-up of diabetics as directed by the family doctor. These techniques were conceived in three moments: firstly, to explain the objectives of the research and to clarify any doubts about it, at the same time as the form was filled in with general personal data: sex, age, skin colour, cultural level and occupation. In addition, questions related to their disease were askedabout their family history, family history family history, comorbidityassociated, complications, lifestyles: smoking, alcoholism, sedentary lifestyle, inadequate diet, glycaemic control and economic situation. Depending on the case, the other instruments were applied at a second and third moment or on different days (Annexes 4 and 5).The stress validation scale, which is an adaptation validated by Cuban authors and approved by MINSAP, was always applied first. It was suggested to follow this order considering the questions that precede and the theme related to stress and family functioning, given the coexistence of interdependence and the need not to suggest or stimulate responses that would lead to bias in the results obtained. For further clarification, the questions for each item were noted and all data were triangulated. Finally, each patient was given the Family Functioning Assessment Test. FF-SIL (appendix 5). This instrument evaluated family functioning (systemic relational dynamics between the members of a family), through the perception of one of the members. It is a simple, low-cost instrument that is easy to understand for any level of education. The test was applied to diabetic patients to obtain their vision of family functioning, and can be self-administered or not. The variables it evaluates are: 1- Cohesion: (items 1 and 8)

1- Cohesion: (items 1 and 8)

2- Harmony (items 2 and 13).

3- Communication (Items 5 and 11).

4- Adaptability (items 6 and 10).

5- Affectivity: (items 4 and 14).

6- Role (items 3 and 9).

7- Permeability (items 7 and 12).mode of application: The subject made an assessment of each proposed statement and responded according to the frequency alternatives presented.
Almost always5 points

Many times4 points

Sometimes3 points

Rarely2 points

Hardly ever1 point

The final score was obtained from the sum of the points per item. The result obtained allowed the family to be placed in one of the following categories:

70 to 57Functional family

From 56 to 43Moderately functional family

From 42 to 28Dysfunctional family

From 27 to 14Severely dysfunctional family

It was pertinent to consider the need for a qualitative analysis of the results in addition to the quantitative analysis proposed by the technique. After collecting all the information, the qualitative technique of data triangulation was used to establish regularities, strengths and weaknesses.

Ethical considerations: Informed consent was requested as a bioethical principle of the research as mentioned above. The information obtained was handled confidentially with the commitment that it would only be used for scientific purposes. (Annex 1).

ANALYSIS OF THE RESULTS

Table 1 in appendix 6 shows the distribution of diabetic patients according to age and sex, where it was observed that 32 females predominated for 54.24%, i.e. more than half of the sample. On the other hand, the age group with the highest incidence was 75-79 years with 18 cases for 30.51%, followed by 70-74 years with 15 cases for 25.42%. Hence, 33 patients are grouped in this age group (70 to 79 years), representing 55.93% of the entire sample, which can be considered a slight majority. Table 2 shows the distribution of patients according to socio-demographic variables in appendix 7. The predominance of white skin colour was found with 52, representing 88.13%; with no schooling, schooling predominated in 18 patients for 30.51%, followed by primary schooling with 16 for 27.12% and in third place were the five cases with secondary schooling for 8.47%.According to occupation, 22 housewives occupied the first place for 37.29%, followed by 20 self-employed workers for 33.90% and nine state workers representing 15.25% of the patients studied. Table 3, appendix 8 shows the distribution of diabetic patients according to clinical characteristics, where it was observed that 38 patients with a history of diabetes predominated, representing 64.41%, i.e. the majority. Obesity and primary hyperlipoproteinaemia were the most prevalent associated comorbidities, reported in 40 patients (67.80%), while arterial hypertension was found in 23 cases (38.98%), so it can be estimated that in this series there is approximately one hypertensive for every two obese diabetics with primary hyperlipoproteinaemia.

The distribution of diabetics in the study according to lifestyle determinants and gender is shown in Table 4, Appendix 9. From this table it could be determined that stress was present in the totality of the sample, inadequate diet in 46 cases for 77.97%, which is equivalent to the great majority, sedentary lifestyle in 34 for 57.63%, and 17 patients (28.81%) were found to have a history of alcoholism. In addition, in the sample of these diabetic smokers, severe smokers predominated, with 43, or 72.88%, reported as such.Table 5 in annex 10 shows the distribution of diabetic patients according to family functioning, where a predominance of functional families was found in 36 cases for 61.02%, however, 16 are moderately functional for 27.12%, five are dysfunctional for 8.47% and two are severely dysfunctional for 3.39%. Hence, the minority (seven) were estimated to be severely dysfunctional families for 11.86%. This representation can be seen in Figure 1 in Annex 10.Table 6 in appendix 11 shows the distribution of diabetic patients according to lifestyle determinants and glycaemic control, showing how t h e incidence of stress affected all patients: 25 with severe lack of control (42.37%) and 28 with slight lack of control (47.45%). These two categories accounted for almost all the patients studied, 53, representing 89.83% of the sample.

The other lifestyle determinant that predominated in second place was inadequate diet, with 25 having severe lack of control (42.37%) and 21 with slight lack of control (35.59%).

Furthermore, in a general sense, in the 25 cases with severe lack of control, the presence of severe smoking was identified for 42.37% of the sample. Stress, inadequate diet and severe smoking were therefore detected in all patients with severe lack of control.

Complications are shown in Table 7, Annex 12, according to lifestyle determinants. Stress and inadequate diet were present in all complications. Alcoholism was evident in all cases with nephropathy, heart disease and retinopathy, as well as sedentary lifestyles in cases of foot ulcers, retinopathy, neuropathy and heart disease.On the other hand, smoking also affected all patients with complications. The highest incidence for diabetic foot was found in the five severe smokers for 8.47%, the three patients with retinopathies and retinopathies for 5.08%, in the 19 patients with neuropathies for 32.20% and in 28 with heart disease for 47.45%.

Table 8, which appears in appendix 13, shows the distribution of diabetic patients according to economic situation and glycaemic control, showing the general predominance of the economic situation classified as high in 26 patients for 44.06%, followed by medium in 11 cases for 18.64% and medium-high in nine for 15.25%. Hence, it was possible to estimate a predominance of high to medium economic situation, with 46 patients in these categories (77.96%), i.e. the majority.

It was observed that in severe dyscontrol the highest incidence was of a medium-low salary in six cases for 10.16%. However, in the 25 patients with severe lack of control, it was possible to estimate the prevalence of a medium to high economic average, as 15.60%, which is more than half, reflect this, for 25.42% of the total sample. A significant relationship was established between economic situation and glycaemic control (p=0.03).

Table 1, which shows the distribution of subjects according to age and sex, the results obtained are similar to those reported by Nina Flores,[53] at the Goyeneche Hospital, where 75.76% of type 2 diabetic patients are over 60 years of age and 83.33% are female, and to Colman et al, [13] in determinants of health in a primary care population, whose data reflect a predominance of diabetics aged 60 years and over (33%) and of the female sex, this behaviour being explained by the fact that women were the ones who attended consultations the most.

Buichia Sombra et al, [54] when analysing the determinants of health and risk of type 2 diabetes in adults from native populations from social theory, it is shown that moderate to vigorous physical activity in crop work is a protective factor for type 2 diabetes in Pima indigenous men from Sonora, and in the case of women, it is suggested that Yoreme-Mayo women continue to play a traditional role by carrying out activities to maintain the household and raise children; these socio-demographic characteristics place this native group in a situation of inequality and poverty, that is, at risk.

With regard to the predominance of the female sex, we also agree with other authors such as Saire Rondon et al.,[55] Rodríguez Ordoñez et al.[48] and Guerra de Campos et al, [30] whose studies determined a percentage of 52.78%, 58.8% and 80% for each one, but differed from them in the age groups, since it was found that 27.78% of the first case were between 31 and 40 years of age; for the second, between 46 and 65 years of age, 58.8% and for the third, 34% responded that they were between 51 and 55 years of age.

Similarly, in the Jipijapa canton,[56] women accounted for 59.16% and in six municipalities in the department of Cortés,[18] by sex in 2014, women had the highest number of new cases of type 2 diabetes mellitus. When assessing age, the data are close to those reported by Sánchez Ramírez et al,[31] in diabetic older adults at the Aguas Frías Health Centre in Medellín, in whose study population a greater number of patients were found between the ages of 65 and 80 years for both sexes. On the other hand, there are no similarities with Gómez Medina,[18] the age range with the highest incidence of DM 2 is 50-59 years, followed by the range 60 years and over; with Solórzano Segovia et al.,[46] 53% of the participants in the study were men nor with Layton Ulloa,[12] in obese diabetic adults 53.39% (n=63) were men and the average age was 53 years for both men and women.

It is the author's opinion that the predominance of older age could be related to the high rates of older adults in the municipality, which is one of the oldest in the province and in the country, which is due to the process of demographic transition in Cuba, and with regard to the female sex, it could be because women tend to seek health services more diligently, as they are more busy and are not subject to as many prejudices as men.

When distributing the sample according to socio-demographic variables as illustrated **in table 2**, the predominance of white skin colour does not coincide with research on socio-economic determinants of diabetes mellitus in a context of inequalities in the Brazilian Northeast,[57] where 74.3% were of the parda/prieta race or others and from Rodríguez Plasencia et al.,[1] on social determinants of health in relation to prevention of diabetic foot in the Belén Hospital, Trujillo, 55.0% are mestizo.

Authors such as Gómez Medina[18] and Santana Suarez et al.,[42] report that this disease has a hereditary tendency and occurs more frequently in the following racial or ethnic groups: [18,42] African Americans, Alaskan Natives, American Indians, Asian Americans, Hispanics or Latinos, Native Hawaiians and Pacific Islanders. Similarly, Layton Ulloa,[12] does not agree with Layton Ulloa, since 95.8% (n=113) of the patients were of mixed race, 3.4% (n=4) were Caucasian and 0.8% (n=1) were Afro-Colombian. By sex, a greater predominance of mestizo ethnicity was observed in women.

When assessing schooling, the findings are similar to those reported in the health centres of Jipijapa, Los Rosales and El Carmen canton,[56] where the level of education was 68.59% and to Pereira da Silva de Carvalho et al.,[57] in Brazil, where 39.4% had less schooling (illiterate/incomplete elementary school), so that these people were almost four times more likely to develop DM. However, this differs from Saire Rondon et al.,[55] which concludes that 58.33% of patients have secondary education followed by primary education at 33.33%. Likewise, Rodríguez Ordoñez et al.[48] and Nina Flores,[53] found that the highest percentage of secondary education was 47.1% (n 40) and 48.48% respectively.

The data are not in line with: Sánchez Ramírez et al.,[31] only 80% of older adults have completed primary school; from Guerra de Campos et al.,[30] as for men 19% reported having studied primary and high school and 31% of women, primary school and from Rodríguez Plasencia et al.,[1] 30.0% have higher education.

Analysing the occupation variable, the result corresponds to the work on social determinants of type 2 diabetes mellitus in users of the Zaragoza Community Family Health Unit,[30] where according to the characterisation of the respondents in the rural area 58% are housewives followed by 29% shopkeepers and in the urban area, 59% are also housewives and in the Goyeneche Hospital,[53] 59.09% of patients are housewives.

On the other hand, the results differ from: Rodríguez Ordoñez et al.,[48] 64.7% of the users with type II diabetes mellitus are either state or private workers; from Pereira da Silva de Carvalho et al.,[57] of the participants from the state, 39.1% were unemployed; Sanchez Ramirez et al.,[31] 86% work in farm work and Rodriguez Plasencia et al.,[1] 21.3% have a casual and independent work status,Similarly it differs from Layton Ulloa,[12] a s the highest percentage of cases (66.1%) had a university degree and 18% were tradesmen, followed by patients with business administration positions (17%) and home-based (10%).

It is inferred that the higher prevalence of housewives as a profession is related to the predominance of the female sex in the sample and to the fact that women have historically been the ones who have taken care of the household. White skin colour coincides with that determined in the municipality, as the population most frequently dispensed is that which calls itself white.

Table 3 shows that diabetic patients with a family history of the disease and with obesity as an associated comorbidity were the most frequent, coinciding with the Colombian study at the Aguas Frías Health Centre,[31] , which found that 32% of older adults had a family history of the disease through their father, 25% through their mother, 14% through their sister, 11% through their grandparents and only 18% were unaware of this. In addition, 58% of the patients have a degree of obesity. This is similar to the findings of Pin Baque et al.,[5] where family history of diabetes in the first and second degree of consanguinity accounted for 52.7% and overweight/obesity for 52.5%, and with results from the Zaragoza Community Family

Health Unit,[30] regarding family members with diabetes. Mellitus Type 2, respondents indicated that 49% have family members with Type 2 Diabetes Mellitus and 46% do not, A similar result was reported in a study carried out in a health care centre in Bucaramanga in which the relationship between social determinants and the evolution of diabetes mellitus in obese adults undergoing bariatric surgery was established. 72.9% of the subjects had a family history of obesity and diabetes (n=86) and 60% had a personal history of dyslipidaemia. [12]

The result found is not related to that reported by Nina Flores,[53] in Arequipa, since 66.67% of patients have arterial hypertension as a background followed by 25.76% with gastritis and 15.15% with osteoarticular diseases. Neither does it coincide with the result of Sotolongo Arró,[58] arterial hypertension was the most frequent associated disease with 86.0 %, nor with that of Ovalle-Luna et al, [59] liver cirrhosis, anaemia or haemoglobinopathies and cancer were determined.The author is of the opinion that both family history of diabetes mellitus and obesity are risk factors strongly associated with the diagnosis of this disease and that is why they were found in a higher percentage in the sample studied. The results corresponding to the distribution of diabetic patients according to lifestyle determinants and sex (**Table 4**) differ from articles such as those of: Colman et al.,[13] who when linking the various risk factors with the variable sex found 67% for inadequate diet and sedentary lifestyle in the female and 33% for the same variables in the male sex and Layton Ulloa,[12] 49.2% of the subjects indicated that the frequency of physical activity was sometimes with the female sex having the highest percentage of people who did not perform any type of activity followed by the factor balanced diet never, 40.7% (n=48). Nor does it resemble the findings of: Morales Arévalo,[26] in Pumacahua-Arequipa, it is observed that the great majority of patients are overweight in 52.5%; de Melo Pérez,[43] in the physical exercise dimension, 67.50% present a regular level and in nutrition, 61.25% also present this level and de Alvarado Magallanes,[60] regarding the consumption of alcohol, 60% do so. 1 time or more per week and 67% drink 3 or more alcoholic beverages on each occasion. Likewise, the result is also unrelated to the findings of Katherine Melissa et al, [22] in lifestyles in patients with type 2 diabetes mellitus in times of pandemic COVID-19, it can be seen that 44.6% (n=70) sometimes manage stress, followed by 41.4% (n=65) with frequent stress management and with Palacios Pintado,[61] regarding the risk factors studied it can be observed that BMI greater than 25 represents the highest percentage (obesity with 49.2% and overweight with 35.6%), which means that 84.8% of the diabetic patients studied have this risk factor present.This means that 84.8% of the diabetic patients studied have this risk factor present. The data obtained are not close to any of the results of the research assessed and it is the author's opinion that this is a finding of the present study and could be related to the increase in the stressors of the current situation and to the increase in smoking, especially among the female sex. The predominance of functional families as shown in **Table 5** does not coincide directly with any of the bibliographies reviewed, but is related to that reported by Astolingon Vela et al.,[47] where it can be seen that in the dimension of family relationships, which evaluates the degree of communication and free expression as well as the degree of interaction within the family, 57.5% (92) of older adults with type II diabetes mellitus have a medium level, followed by 28.8% (46) with a high level and 13.8% (22) with a low level.

Pérez Rodríguez et al. state that family support has an impact on the disease, its evolution and outcome, so that it is a fundamental element in developing health and self-care behaviours, as well as the patient's adherence to medical treatment. Adequate family functionality allows for adaptability, solidarity, affection and the ability to solve problems. [11]

In a study on family support and adherence to treatment in patients with type II diabetes mellitus,[48] showed that regular instrumental support predominated, 29.4%; regular emotional, 29.4%; regular spiritual, 42.4% and regular economic, 38.8%. Other authors, such as Roldán Cedeño et. al.[56] and Solórzano Segovia et. al.[46] , when analysing family structure, found that 82.72% had extended families in the first case and in the second, it was concluded that living with a partner was associated with a better health profile than in the homologous population that did not live with a partner. The data obtained differ from Salvador Bonilla, in family functionality and pharmacological therapeutic adherence in type 2 diabetic patients, in which it is reported that, of the population under study, only 8.3% of the families are functional, while 91.9% present some degree of dysfunctionality, with moderately functional families prevailing with 53.3%, followed by dysfunctional families with 53.3%.30%. [62]The author states that, in the population seen in the study clinic, functional families predominate and that this could explain why a higher percentage of families were found to be functional. Percentage this condition was found in a higher percentage. The predominance of mildly uncontrolled glycaemia, as shown **in table 6**, is similar to the findings in a general hospital in Peru, [63] where 31.2% of patients were overweight and 43.7% obese, with fasting glycaemia > 100 mg/dl 112 (91.8%) subjects without complications and 70 (92,1%) with complications. The result is also in line with Guerra Uriarte et al, [45] where 65.22% of patients had inadequate fasting glycaemia and 76.09% had inadequate postprandial glycaemia; Morales Arévalo,[26] shows that glycaemia levels are elevated in 21 patients (52.5%) and Palacios Pintado,[61] states that there is a relationship between elevated glucose levels, elevated body mass index, elevated abdominal perimeter and elevated triglyceride levels. This result is not related to the research carried out at the Bellavista Health Centre,[61] , when assessing the relationship between the risk factors for type II diabetes and lifestyles, since the glucose levels measured in 88 patients (74.6%) were found to be normal (equal to or less than 110) and in only 30 (25.4%) were values higher than this figure. This means that the majority of diabetic patients are under control.The author is of the opinion that the findings are partly related to the difficult economic situation in the country, which means that a diet and medication regimen can be well managed, but it cannot be denied that there is a certain degree of neglect in self-care by those suffering from this pathology. The distribution of diabetic patients according to lifestyle determinants and complications (**Table 7**) shows, in relation to the predominance of diabetic neuropathy, results similar to Sotolongo Arró,[58] in Punta Brava, Cuba, where this was the most frequent complication for 79.3 %, with women standing out (55.3 %) and Asenjo Alarcón et al, [64] in an Andean city in Peru, the frequency of diabetic neuropathy was 36.4% followed by diabetic retinopathy (27.3%). When assessing the determinants, we agree with Valdés Ramos et al.,[65] . Among the seven risk factors associated with cardiovascular complications in diabetic women, smoking was one of the factors that independently increased risk, as demonstrated by multivariate analysis, and with Coronado Balderas,[66] . 65.1% of patients were inactive or sedentary, and with regard to smoking, 60.3% smoked, of which 38.1% had a smoking index <Katherine Melissa et al.[22] and Cebrián Cuenca,[15] state that the increased risk of these complications is due to multiple factors such as limited physical activity, increased sedentary behaviour, limited access to fruit and vegetables and, in

general, increased food insecurity. In addition, it is partially similar to what was observed by Ochoa Anastacio,[67] in which it is shown that 42% of the older adults sometimes do physical activity and 28% almost never, but it differs when determining the associated complications, where there was a predominance of arterial hypertension in 18 patients (50%) and diabetic nephropathy (30%).

However, what was observed in the present investigation differs from studies such as that of the Enrique Ponce Luque Health Centre,[68] 53% of users have suffered from skin ulcers, this complication being the one with the highest incidence and according to the result obtained, 63% occasionally ingest alcoholic beverages and Villacorta Santamato et al, [63] in the group with chronic microvascular complications, nephropathy (48.8%) was the most frequent, and in the macrovascular group, cerebrovascular disease (4.8%), and overweight and obesity were the main risk factors for 43.7%. Nor does it resemble that reported by Santos Quezada[69] who reported diabetic foot as the most frequent associated complication and Ovalle Luna et al.,[59] in Mexico, concluded that foot disease was recorded in 50,635 (17.0 %) of the population.

%) patients, chronic kidney disease (CKD) in 21 605 (7.2 %), and retinopathy in 13 115 (4.4 %).

When analysing the distribution of diabetic patients according to economic status and glycaemic control, as shown in **Table 8**, the results obtained differ from those of Rodríguez Plasencia et al: Rodríguez Plasencia et al.,[1] who states that 50.0% of patients with diabetic foot have a medium socioeconomic level, from Holguín Carrasquilla,[32] 53.49% of diabetic adults show a low economic level and from Roldán Cedeño et al.,[56] 58.63% of users were below the poverty line determining this as a risk factor.

In a systematic review on the social determinants of health in type 2 diabetes, Limón García et al.,[3] , it is stated that a relevant factor in the development of the disease was poor diet, prolonged fasting, high fat intake, excess consumption of meat and ultra-processed foods in the diet that were associated with physical inactivity and low economic status.

The results do not correspond either with the Brazilian study,[57] of the participants 39.4% were classified in the poorest economic class and of these, 49.7% received family allowance; from Peruvian work,[53] 43.94% of patients have a monthly household income of less than one minimum wage and from research in Puno,[7] of the 100% of patients surveyed 59.1% indicated that they have a monthly income of less than 1025 of which 55.2% do not comply with the treatment. Pereira da Silva et al. argue that individuals with low socio-economic status may be more vulnerable to such diseases for several reasons, including psychosocial stress, higher levels of risk behaviour such as sedentary lifestyles and high consumption of higher calorie foods rich in sugar and fat, unhealthy living conditions, poor access to basic sanitation and health services, and reduced opportunity to prevent complications. [57] The prevalence of high economic status does not correspond to any of the articles reviewed by the author and, according to her, could be due to the fact that in the municipality where the research was carried out there is intense commercial activity that determines a certain economic solvency of some social groups and also because the literature reviewed is from developing countries where the studies are limited to populations with medium and low resources, but do not address the affluent class.

CONCLUSIONS

The sample was dominated by women aged 75-79 years, white, unschooled, housewives, with a family history of diabetes mellitus, as well as obesity and primary hyperlipoproteinaemia were the most prevalent associated comorbidities. The social determinants of health that most affected the patients studied were stress, smoking and inadequate diet, which were present in all complications. In addition, there was a general predominance of economic status classified as high.

REFERENCES BIBLIOGRAPHIC

1. Rodríguez Plasencia CB, Villacorta Flores NE. Determinantes sociales de la salud en relación con prevención del pie diabético en el Hospital Belén, Trujillo, 2022 [Thesis]. Peru: Universidad Privada Antenor Orrego; 2023. Available at: http://repositorio.upao.edu.pe/bitstream/20.500.12759/10360/1/REP_CECILIA.ROD RI GUIEZ_NICOLL.VILLACORTA_DETERMINANTS.SOCIAL.pdf

2. Valdés Gómez W, Almirall Sánchez A, Gutiérrez Pérez MÁ. Risk factors for type 2 diabetes mellitus in adolescents. MediSur [Internet]. 2019 [cited 21 Mar 2023];17(3):[approx.8p.]. Available from: http://scielo.sld.cu/pdf/ms/v17n3/1727- 897Xms-17-03-356.pdf.

3. Limón García L, Dominguez SA, Palacios Rodríguez AL. Social determinants of health in type 2 diabetes: a systematic review. Revista Hospitum [Internet]. 2022 [cited 21 Mar 2023];4:[approx.9p.]. Available from: https://www.hospitalquindio.gov.co/hospital/images/banners/Revista_hospital_ospitu m.pdf#page=44.

4. Duarte Acha MY, Ribeiro Zanotti J, Vieira Gomes R, Cruz Hegner C, de Freitas Valbon B. Alterações oftalmológicas em crianças e adolescentes portadores de diabetes mellitus tipo 1 em um Hospital Filantrópico de Vitória-ES. [Internet]. 2020 [cited 21 Mar 2023]:[approx.18p.]. Available from: https://downloads.editoracientifica.org/articles/200901276.pdf.

5. Pin Baque WE, Quevedo Andrade YM. Risk factors of Diabetes Mellitus type II and its relationship to eating disorders in adults [Thesis]. Jipijapa: Unesum; 2023. Available at: http://repositorio.unesum.edu.ec/bitstream/53000/4941/1/PIN%20BAQUE%20WALTE R%20ENRIQUE%20%20%20-20QUEVEDO%20ANDRADE%20YULEXI%20MICHEL.pdf

6. Chavelas S, Luis J. Proyecto de intervención para mejorar el conocimiento sobre la diabetes mellitus tipo 2 en pacientes diagnosticados con esta enfermedad atendidos en el Centro de Salud T-II Ampliación Selene, Tláhuac, Ciudad de México, en el periodo de enero a abril del 2021 [Thesis]. Autonomous Metropolitan University;2022. Available at: https://repositorio.xoc.uam.mx/jspui/handle/123456789/26457

7. Arpita Laruta DR, Centeno Palero AL. Factors associated with dropout Terapéutico en Pacientes con Diabetes Mellitus tipo II de la Red de Salud Puno, 2022 [Thesis]. Huancayo - Peru: Roosevelt University; 2022. Available at: https://repositorio.uroosevelt.edu.pe/bitstream/handle/20.500.14140/1217/TESIS%20 ARPITA%20-%20CENTENO.pdf?sequence=1&isAllowed=y

8. Gómez Baldeón LL, Pacheco Tolentino CK. Factors associated with type II diabetes mellitus in older adults at the Centro de Salud Aparicio Pomares, Huánuco 2021 [Thesis]. Chincha, Ica: Universidad Autónoma de Ica; 2022. Available in: http://repositorio.autonomadeica.edu.pe/handle/autonomadeica/1581

9. Lema Añón C. The revolution of the social determinants of health: right to health and inequality. Yearbook of Philosophy of Law [Internet]. 2020 [cited 21 Mar

2023]:[approx.28p.]. Available from:
https://www.boe.es/biblioteca_juridica/anuarios_derecho/abrir_pdf.php?id=ANU- F2020-10028900317.

10. Karam Calderón MÁ, Castillo Sánchez Y, Moreno Pérez P, Ramírez Durán N, Dubos R. What are the social determinants of health? Journal of Medicine and Research [Internet]. 2021 [cited 21 Mar 2023];7(1):[approx.7p.]. Available from:

https://rmi.diauaemex.com/index.php/numeros/ano-2019/23-que-son-losdeterminantes- social-of-health.

11. Pérez Rodríguez A, Berenguer Gouarnaluses M. Some social determinants and their association with type 2 diabetes mellitus. Medisan [Internet]. 2015 [cited 21 Mar 2023];19(10):[approx.3p.]. Available from:
http://scielo.sld.cu/scielo.php?script=sci_arttext&pid=S1029- 30192015001000012.

12. Layton Ulloa S. Relationship Between Social Determinants and the Evolution of Diabetes Mellitus in Obese Adults Undergoing Bariatric Surgery [Thesis].
Colombia: Universidad de Santander; 2023. Available at:
https://repositorio.udes.edu.co/server/api/core/bitstreams/f9c83072-2027-44bc-a247bcfeba2858d2/content

13. Colman R, Sousa R, Vera N, Encina K, Lezcano L, Romero J, et al. Determinants of health in type II diabetes in an urban centre primary care population, 2019. Scientific Journal Studies and Research [Internet]. 2019 [cited 21 Mar 2023];8:[approx.3p.]. Available from: http://revista.unibe.edu.py/index.php/rcei/article/view/363.

14. Heredia M, Cabriales ECG. Risk of type 2 diabetes mellitus and its determinants. Global Nursing [Internet]. 2022 [cited 21 Mar 2023];21(1):[approx.23p.]. Available from:
https://revistas.um.es/eglobal/article/view/482971/315531.

15. Cebrián Cuenca AM. Social inequalities in the health and control of type 2 diabetes mellitus. Diabetes práctica [Internet]. 2022 [cited 21 Mar 2023];1(Suppl Extr 1):[approx.38p.]. Available from: http://www.diabetespractica.com/files/101/art3.pdf.

16. MINSAP. Programa Nacional de Atención Integral al Diabético. Cuba.2011. p. approx.6p.

17. Health statistical yearbook 2019. [Internet]. Havana: Ministry of Health. Public. Directorate of medical records and health statistics; 2020 [updated May 2020; cited 15/02/21; cited 2021]. Available from: http://bvscuba.sld.cu/anuarioestadistico-de-cuba/

18. Gómez Medina MJ. Desigualdades sociales de la salud en pacientes con diabetes tipo II en seis municipios del departamento de Cortés años 2014 y 2016 [Tesis]. Honduras: Universidad Nacional Autónoma de Honduras; 2019. Available from:
http://www.bvs.hn/TMSP/pdf/TMSP55/pdf/TMSP55.pdf

19. Lorenzo Villena JA. Type 1 diabetes mellitus at school age. Diabetes [Internet]. 2020 [cited 21 Mar 2023];3(27):[approx.18p.]. Available from:
https://www.npunto.es/content/src/pdf-articulo/5ee22d46dd243NPvolumen27-40-57.pdf.

20. Rodríguez-Tenorio Torres R, Orduna Onco Á. Health education programme in the

management of new devices for the control of diabetes in adolescents aged 15-18 years. [Internet]. 2020 [cited 19/05/21]:[approx.6p.].
Available at: https://zaguan.unizar.es/record/96690/files/TAZ-TFG-2020-377.pdf .

21. Bondía J. Artificial pancreas Artificial pancreas. Rev Esp Endocrinol Pediatr [Internet]. 2020 [cited 19/05/21];11(1):[approx.6p.]. Available from: https://www.endocrinologiapediatrica.org/revistas/P1-E33/P1-E33-S2620- A599.pdf. 22. Katherine Melissa LL, Herrera Calderón VP. Lifestyles in patients with type 2 diabetes mellitus in times of pandemic COVID-19. Sapienza: International Journal of Interdisciplinary Studies [Internet]. 2022 [cited 21 Mar 2023];3(8):[approx.8p.]. Available from: https://journals.sapienzaeditorial.com/index.php/SIJIS/article/view/582.

23. Campos Rojas MM, Quintana Padilla TG. Autocuidado y factores condicionantes en el adulto mayor con diabetes mellitus del Centro de Salud Chilca Huancayo 2022 [Thesis]. Peru: Roosevelt University; 2023. Available in: https://repositorio.uroosevelt.edu.pe/bitstream/handle/20.500.14140/1412/TESIS%20 QUINTANA%20-%20CAMPOS.pdf?sequence=1&isAllowed=y

24. Flores Vasquez DS. Study of type 1 diabetes mellitus with ketoacidosis in children for its correct diagnosis and pharmacological treatment [Thesis]. Machala: Universidad Técnica de Machala; 2021. Available at: http://repositorio.utmachala.edu.ec/bitstream/48000/16189/1/E-11893_FLORES%20VASQUEZ%20DERYAN%20SANTIAGO%20.pdf

25. Suero Girardi MN. Quality of life of adolescents with diabetes. University of Flores [Internet]. 2020 [cited 21 Mar 2023];1(5):[approx.20p.]. Available from: https://d1wqtxts1xzle7.cloudfront.net/19115256/calidaddevidauflo_n5v1pp3_22.pdf.

26. Morales Arévalo NJ. Relación entre los niveles de glicemia y comportamiento de estilos de vida en pacientes con Diabetes Mellitus tipo 2 de la localidad de Mateo Pumacahua-Arequipa 2022 [Tesis]. Peru: Universidad Católica de Santa María; 2022. Available at: https://repositorio.ucsm.edu.pe/bitstream/handle/20.500.12920/11899/70.2838.M.pdf ?sequence=1&isAllowed=y

27. Osti ZAT, Lezama JAF. Risk Factors Associated with Type 2 Diabetes Mellitus in Adolescents. Mexican Journal of Medical Research ICSA [Internet]. 2020 [cited 15/06/21];8(15):[approx.7p.]. Available from: https://repository.uaeh.edu.mx/revistas/index.php/MJMR/article/view/3932/6995.

28. Ramírez Rivera NK. Calidad de vida en pacientes con diabetes mellitus tipo II, centro de salud Bambil Deshecho, Santa Elena, 2022 [Thesis]. La Libertad: Santa Elena Peninsula State University; 2023. Available in: https://repositorio.upse.edu.ec/bitstream/46000/9568/1/UPSE-TEN-2023-0027.pdf

29. Alejandria Quispe YY. Sociodemographic characteristics and lifestyles in adults with Diabetes Mellitus. Centro de salud Morro Solar-Jaén-Perú 2021 [Thesis]. Peru: National University of Cajamarca; 2022. Available in: https://repositorio.unc.edu.pe/handle/20.500.14074/4924

30. Guerra de Campos SE, Aragón de Melara AB. Social determinants of type 2 diabetes mellitus in users aged 35-55 years consulting in the Family Health Community Unit of Zaragoza February to September 2019 [Thesis]. El Salvador: University of El Salvador; 2019. Disponible en: https://docs.bvsalud.org/biblioref/2020/12/1140671/289-11106299.pdf

31. Sanchez Ramirez LK, Onofre Torres MJ. Lifestyles and their influence on type II diabetes mellitus, in older adults of the Aguas Frias Health Center of Medellin Ventanas, Los Ríos, October 2018-April 2019 [Thesis]. Babahoyo: Universidad Técnica de Babahoyo; 2019. Available from: http://dspace.utb.edu.ec/bitstream/handle/49000/5852/P-UTB-FCS-ENF-000130.pdf?sequence=1&isAllowed=y.

32. Holguín Carrasquilla MP. Autocuidado y complicaciones del adulto diabético en la población del Subcentro Tipo C de San Rafael [Thesis]. Ecuador: PuceseEscuela de Enfermería; 2022. Available at: https://repositorio.pucese.edu.ec/bitstream/123456789/3245/1/Holgu%c3%adn%20C arrasquilla%20Melanie%20Paola.pdf

33. Arzate J, Rangel J. Social determinants of health. A sociological argument. In: Porvenir E, editor ^editors. Vulnerability, health and social policies. [Internet]. First eclicirin ed. Mexico: Instituto de Investigaciones Sociales; 2021.

p. approx. 27p. Available at: http://ri.uaemex.mx/bitstream/handle/20.500.11799/111906/DeterminantesSacia.pdf?sequence=1&isAllowed=y
34. Robles MJ, Gómez Bermúdez J. Análisis de los determinantes sociales de la salud que intervienen o influyen en el estado de salud de una comunidad [Thesis]. Colombia: Simón Bolivar University; 2021.

35. Hernandez-Rincon EH. The social determinants of child malnutrition in Colombia as seen from family medicine. Medwave [Internet]. 2020 [cited 21 Mar 2023];20(2):[approx.11p.]. Available from: https://www.researchgate.net/profile/Erwin-Hernandez-

Rincon/publication/339953732_Los_determinantes_sociales_de_de_la_desnutricion_in_Colom bia_vistos_desde_desicina_familiar/links/5e6f961a299bf12e23cbd3 b2/Los_determinantes_sociales_de_la_desnutricion_in_Colombia-vistos-desdela- medicina-familiar.pdf.
36. Prado Cuadros T, Sermeño Palacios CL. Social determinants of the abandonment of exclusive breastfeeding in term infants under 6 months at the Margomarca Health Center in San Juan de Lurigancho, 2017 [Thesis]. Peru: Maria Auxiliadora University; 2018. Available at: https://repositorio.uma.edu.pe/bitstream/handle/20.500.12970/165/Tesis%20Abandon o%20Lactancia%20Materna.pdf?sequence=1&isAllowed=y
37. Treacy M. The social determinants of health in the neoliberal era: a political economy approach to inequalities. Essays in Economics [Internet]. 2021 [cited 21 Mar 2023];31(58):[approx.23p.]. Available from: http://www.scielo.org.co/scielo.php?script=sci_arttext&pid=S261965732021000100134

38. Espada López J, Hernández Clemente JC. Health indicators and social and structural determinants in the Spanish health environment. A propósito de la crisis económica 2008-2014 [Thesis]. Spain: Universidad Autónoma de Madrid;

2022. Available at:

https://acmspublicaciones.revistabarataria.es/wpcontent/uploads/2023/05/14-Espada- Clemente-Indicadores-de-salud-2019-2023pp157-167.pdf

39. Moreno Gómez MdM, Hernández Rincón EH, Ayala Escudero A, Correal Muñoz CA. Teaching and learning about social determinants of health in the region of the Americas. Educación Médica Superior [Internet]. 2021 [cited 21 Mar 2023];35(3):[approx.25p.]. Available from: http://scielo.sld.cu/scielo.php?script=sci_arttext&pid=S0864-21412021000300018.

40. Peña S, Franciss J. Consumption of fruits and vegetables as a protector of oral health and social determinants of health in people older than 15 years, Peru-2018 [Thesis]. Peru: Universidad Peruana Cayetano Heredia; 2021. Available in:

https://190.116.48.43/bitstream/handle/20.500.12866/9535/Consumo_SalasPena_Jo nathan.pdf?sequence=1&isAllowed=y

41. Pérez Martínez GB. Social determinants of health: An overview in Mexico and Chiapas. Revista Anales de Medicina Universitaria [Internet]. 2022 [cited 21 Mar 2023];1(02):[approx.7p.]. Available from: http://www.revistas.unach.mx/index.php/revanales/article/view/30.

42. Santana Suarez JC, Licoa Zavala JK. Comorbidities associated with type II diabetes mellitus: causes, consequences and prevalence in older adults [Thesis]. Jipijapa: Unesum; 2023. Available at:

http://repositorio.unesum.edu.ec/bitstream/53000/4954/1/Santana%20Suarez%20Juli ssa%20Celestina%20-%20Licoa%20Zavala%20Julissa%20Katherine.pdf

43. Melo Pérez MJ. Influencia de los estilos de vida en la salud de pacientes adultos con diabetes mellitus tipo II en el Hospital René Toche Groppo Chincha Alta2017 [Thesis]. Peru: Universidad Inca Garcilaso de La Vega; 2020. Available at:

http://repositorio.uigv.edu.pe/bitstream/handle/20.500.11818/5216/TESIS_MEL O%20 P%c3%89REZ.pdf?sequence=1&isAllowed=y

44. Daufi Subirats MC, Romera Liébana L. Is diabetes mellitus a social disease? Diabetes práctica [Internet]. 2020 [cited 21 Mar 2023];11(032020):[approx.34p.]. Available from: http://www.diabetespractica.com/files/1603725214.dp_11-3.pdf#page=5.

45. Guerra Uriarte JEN, López Cáceres PL. Influence of lifestyles, sociodemographic and clinical characteristics on glycemic control in patients with type 2 diabetes mellitus. Centro de Salud 4 de Octubre, Socabaya-Arequipa 2022 [Thesis]. Peru: Catholic University of Santa Maria; 2022. Available in:

https://repositorio.ucsm.edu.pe/bitstream/handle/20.500.12920/11657/70.2787.M.pdf?sequence =1&isAllowed=y

46. Solórzano Segovia J, Segovia Medina M, Delgado Armijos M, Delgado Armijos

E. Social determinants of health and risks of type 2 diabetes mellitus. Revista Científica Biomédica Higía de la Salud [Internet]. 2020 [cited 21 Mar 2023];3(2):[approx.11p.]. Available from: https://revistas.itsup.edu.ec/index.php/Higia/article/view/469/640.

47. Astolingon Vela RI, Vilca Lucana LK. Family climate and depression in older adults with Type II diabetes mellitus. Programa del adulto mayor-centro de salud de Morales. May to October 2021 [Thesis]. Peru: Universidad Nacional San Martin; 2021. Available in:https://tesis.unsm.edu.pe/bitstream/11458/4278/1/ENFERMER%c3%8dA%20-%20Rosa%20Isabel%20Astoling%c3%b3n%20Vela%20%26%20Leidy%20Kalen%20Vilca%20Lucana.pdf

48. Rodríguez Ordoñez LC, De La Cruz Taipe J. Family support and adherence to treatment of type II diabetes mellitus in users of a health centre [Thesis]. Peru: University Peruana Los Andes; 2021. Available at: https://repositorio.upla.edu.pe/handle/20.500.12848/2319

49. Roca R. Topics in Internal Medicine. 5th ed. Diseases of the circulatory system. Havana: Ecimed; 2017.

50. Álvarez Sintes R, Hernández Cabrera G, Báster Moro JC, García Núñez RD. Medicina General Integral. Volume II. Third edition. Editorial Ciencias Médicas. 2014. Havana. Cuba.

51. Banting F. G. History of diabetes [Internet] [updated 2015; cited 5 Jun 2022]. [Internet]. [cited].AvailableAt: www.wmu.org.uy/publicaciones/libros/historicos/dm/cap1.pdf.

52. Smoking. Consumption of products made wholly or partly with tobacco. World Health Organization [Internet] 2016. [cited 20 Mar 2022]. WHO:Smoking. [Internet].[cited]. Available from: https://www.who.int/topics/tobacco/es/.

53. Nina Flores KC. Association between social determinants and lifestyles of patients with Diabetes Mellitus Type 2 Hospital Goyeneche, Arequipa 2020 [Thesis]. Peru: Universidad Católica de Santa María; 2020. Available at: https://repositorio.ucsm.edu.pe/handle/20.500.12920/10151

54. Buichia Sombra FG, Miranda Cota GA. Social determinants of health and risk of Type 2 diabetes in adults from native populations, approaches from social theory. Journal of the Academy [Internet]. 2021 [cited 14 Mar 2023] (4):[approx.24p.]. Available from:

https://journalacademy.net/index.php/revista/article/view/45/41.

55. Saire Rondon FM, Takahashi Moreno YM. Eating habits and type II diabetes mellitus in patients attending the health post Union-Puerto Maldonado, 2019 [Thesis]. Puerto Maldonado: Universidad Nacional Amazónica de Madre De Dios; 2021. Available at: https://repositorio.unamad.edu.pe/bitstream/handle/20.500.14070/698/004-1-9-040.pdf?sequence=1&isAllowed=y

56. Roldán Cedeño CP, Cedeño Zambrano AP. Socioeconomic determinants and their influence on the level of risk of foot complications in people with Diabetes mellitus 2 in the health centres of Jipijapa, Los Rosales and El Roldán Cedeño CP, Cedeño Zambrano AP.

Carmen, en el periodo noviembre 2020-agosto 2021 [Thesis]. Ecuador: Pontificia Universidad Católica del Ecuador; 2021. Available at: http://repositorio.puce.edu.ec/bitstream/handle/22000/19399/Tesis%20final%20ADRI

ANA%20CEDENO%20Y%20CINTHIA%20ROLDAN.pdf?sequence=1&isAllowed=y

57. Pereira da Silva de Carvalho S, Sobreira de Carvalho Barreto MN, de Souza NP, Cabral de Lira PI, Pessoa Cesse EÂ. Determinantes socioeconômicos do diabetes mellitus em um contexto de desigualdades no nordeste brasileiro. Revista Eletrônica Acervo Saúde [Internet]. 2021 [cited 14 Mar 2023];13(5):[approx.9p.].
Available at: https://acervomais.com.br/index.php/saude/article/view/6863/4561.

58. Sotolongo Arró O. Chronic complications and associated diseases in older adults with type 2 diabetes mellitus in Punta Brava, Cuba from January to June 2019. Cuban Journal of Endocrinology [Internet]. 2022 [cited 14 Mar 2023];33(1):[aprox.11p.]. Available at: http://scielo.sld.cu/scielo.php?pid=S156129532022000100003&script=sci_arttext&tl ng=pt.
59. Ovalle-Luna OD, Jiménez-Martínez IA, Rascón-Pacheco RA, Gómez-Díaz RA, Valdez-González AL, Gamiochipi-Cano M, et al. Prevalence of complications of diabetes and associated comorbidities in family medicine at the Mexican Institute of Diabetes.
Social Security. Gaceta medica de Mexico [Internet]. 2019 [cited 14 Mar 2023];155(1):[approx.9p.]. Available from:
https://www.scielo.org.mx/scielo.php?script=sci_arttext&pid=S00163813201900010 0030.
60. Alvarado Magallanes AE. Behavioural risk factors in older adults with type II diabetes mellitus. Hospital general Dr. León Becerra Camacho, Milagro 2022 [Thesis]. La Libertad: Santa Elena Peninsula State University; 2023.
Available at: https://repositorio.upse.edu.ec/bitstream/46000/9566/1/UPSE-TEN- 2023-0001.pdf

61. Palacios Pintado EB. Relationship between risk factors for Type I diabetes and Type II diabetes. II and lifestyles in patients attending the Centro de Salud Bellavista 2019 [Thesis]. Peru: National University of Callao; 2020. Available at:
http://repositorio.unac.edu.pe/handle/20.500.12952/5343

62. Salvador Bonilla IA. Family functionality and pharmacological therapeutic adherence in type 2 diabetic patients in a primary health care unit [Thesis]. Ecuador: Universidad Técnica de Ambato...; 2022. Available at:
http://repositorio.uta.edu.ec/bitstream/123456789/34913/1/salvador_bonilla_ivonne_a lexandratesis_funcionalidad_familiar_y_adherencia_terap%c3%a9utica .pdf 63.
Villacorta Santamato J, Hilario Huapaya N, Inolopú Cucche J, Terrel Gutierrez

L, Labán Hijar R, Del Aguila J, et al. Factors associated with chronic complications of type 2 diabetes mellitus in patients in a general hospital of the Peruvian Social Health Insurance.
Annals of the Faculty of Medicine [Internet]. 2020 [cited 14 Mar 2023];81(3):[approx.7p.].
Available from:
http://www.scielo.org.pe/scielo.php?script=sci_arttext&pid=S1025558320200003003 08.
64. Asenjo-Alarcón JA, Oblitas-Gonzales A. Chronic microvascular complications in users with type 2 diabetes mellitus in an Andean city of Peru. Revista de Salud Pública [Internet]. 2022 [cited 20 Jun 2023];24(3):[approx.8p.].
Available at:
http://www.scielo.org.co/scielo.php?script=sci_arttext&pid=S012400642022000300201.

65. Valdés Ramos ER, Valdés Bencosme ER, Valdés Bencosme NN. Risk factors associated with cardiovascular complications in middle-aged women with type 2 diabetes mellitus. Cuban Journal of Endocrinology [Internet].
2020 [cited 14 Mar 2023];31(2):[approx.14p.]. Available from:

http://scielo.sld.cu/scielo.php?script=sci_arttext&pid=S1561-29532020000200006.

66. Coronado Balderas DA. Lifestyle associated with complications in patients with diabetes mellitus 2 [Thesis]. Mexico: Benemérita Universidad Autónoma de Puebla 2021. Available at: https://repositorioinstitucional.buap.mx/handle/20.500.12371/13626

67. Ochoa Anastacio ME. Modifiable factors that influence the presence of Complications in Older Adults with Diabetes Mellitus Type II in the Lupita Nolivos Older Adults Club April-September 2019 [Thesis]. Ecuador: Universidad Estatal de Milagro; 2021. Available in:

https://repositorio.unemi.edu.ec/bitstream/123456789/5746/1/MARIA%20ELENA%20
OCHOA%20ANASTACIO.pdf

68. Cabezas Bolaños DL, Montoya Vélez AB. Lifestyles and their influence on the development of health complications in adult patients with type 2 diabetes mellitus.
2 attended at the Enrique Ponce Luque Health Centre December 2022-May 2023 [Thesis]. Peru: Babahoyo: UTB-FCS; 2023. Available at:
http://dspace.utb.edu.ec/bitstream/handle/49000/14314/TIC-UTB-FCS-ER-
000005.pdf?sequence=1&isAllowed=y

69. Santos Quezada AM. Risk factors and complications in type 2 diabetes mellitus in patients older than 40 years Hospital Nacional Dos de Mayo, 2018-2019 [Thesis]. Peru: Universidad Privada San Juan Bautista; 2020. Available at:
https://repositorio.upsjb.edu.pe/handle/20.500.14308/2467

ANNEXES

ANNEX 1: GUIDE FOR CONDUCTING THE DOCUMENTARY ANALYSIS.

Objective: To collect information and data of interest to the study for the characterisation of the diabetic patients selected in the research sample according to clinical and socio-demographic variables.

Tasks:

1. Review of the Family Doctor Programme and the National Programme for Integrated Diabetic Care.
2. Documentary review of the family records of the health area.

3. Documentary review of the individual medical records of t h e patients in the sample.
4. Emptying of the collected data into a data file.

Aspects to be taken into account:

Family Doctor's Programme and the National Programme for Comprehensive Diabetic Care: objectives related to the subject, promotion, prevention and work with risk groups, as well as indications for the comprehensive care of type 2 diabetic patients.

-Family medical records. Socio-demographic variables

-Sex.Female Male

-Age

-Level of schooling

• Out of school

• Primary

• Secondary

• Skilled worker

• Medium technician

• Pre-university

• University

-Occupation

• State worker

• Self-employed

• Retired

• Housewife

• Carer of another elderly person or sick relative

• Patient being cared for by a relative or other person

-Family history of diabetes

   No previous history

41

With antecedents. Specify which: mother, father, grandparents and siblings.

-Individual case histories: Clinical and epidemiological variables

-Skin colour. White Not white -Associated comorbidity.
Arterial Hypertension. Yes No

Obesity. Yes No Primary HyperlipoproteinaemiasYes No
History of Ischaemic Heart DiseaseYes No Chronic Kidney Disease Yes No
Others, which ones

-Complications

Diabetic foot ulcer.Yes No Diabetic retinopathy.

Yes No Diabetic neuropathy Yes No Nephropathy. Yes No Heart disease Yes No
Other, mention which one.

ANNEX 2. SEMI-STRUCTURED INDIVIDUAL QUESTIONNAIRE FOR TYPE 2 DIABETICS. CLINIC 14-32

Objective: to identify data of interest for the study associated with their way of life and lifestyle, as well as the information they have about their illness and their opinions about it. Aimed at patients selected for the study.

Venue: patients' home Time: from 2.00 PM onwards

Questionnaire for type 2 diabetics. Clinic 14-32

As you have already been informed, a research is being carried out to study the biological, psychological and social factors that are most affecting diabetic patients in the health area. You were selected to participate after giving your consent and you are reminded that your answers are confidential so your name will not appear in any document but the number assigned to you.
For your cooperation, thank you very much1
Assigned number

You will then be asked for your general personal details in order to fill in the form:

1. Sex Female Male

2. Age

3. Skin colour: White Black 4.-Schooling level
Out of school Primary Secondary Skilled worker

Medium technician Pre-university   University

5. Current occupation: State worker Self-employed Retired Homemaker Caregiver of another elderly or sick relative

Patient being cared for by a relative or other person **Questions related to their illness:**
6. Do you have family members with diabetes? Yes No

6- b. If yes, please state who: mother, father, grandparents and/or siblings

7- Do you suffer from any other diseases besides diabetes? Please list them.
Arterial Hypertension. Yes No Obesity.Yes No

Primary Hyperlipoproteinaemias Yes No History of Ischaemic Heart Disease Yes No Chronic Kidney Disease Yes No
Others, which ones

8- Please tell us if you have any complications or complications due to diabetes, which one(s)?

Diabetic foot ulcer. Yes No Diabetic retinopathy. Yes No Diabetic neuropathy Yes No
Nephropathy. Yes No Heart disease Yes No
Other, mention which one.

9. In relation to your daily habits please answer:

9.1.a. Do you smoke or have you ever smoked?

Smoker Yes. No.Ex-smoker: Yes. No

9.1.b. If yes, please state the number of cigarettes you smoke or used to smoke per day:
Less than 5 cigarettes per day Light smoker 6 to 15 cigarettes per day Moderate smoker
More than 16 cigarettes a day. Severe smoker

10. Do you consume alcoholic beverages? Yes No

10.b. If yes, please explain how often you do it and how much you consume.

11. a. Do you attend the grandparents' circle?YesNo

11. b. Do you do morning gymnastics at home? Yes No

11. c. Do you walk or walk up and down stairs several times a week as part of your daily
activity? Yes No

11. d. Do you plan to exercise two or three times a week?Yes No
11.e. Answer honestly whether you consider yourself to be sedentary. Explain your reasons:

12. What are the main foods you eat every day for a week? Explain the elaboration.

13. How well do you feel your glycaemia is controlled most of the time?

Well controlled Slightly out of control Severe lack of control Please give your opinion.

14. In relation to their economic situation an estimate needs to be made to calculate the
average per person.

With whom do you live? And what salary does each of them have? Calculate and tick as
appropriate below:

15. Please express your opinion on: What does it mean to you to be diabetic? Please explain
your answer.

16. Express any difficulties or concerns regarding your illness.

Thank you very much for your cooperation!

ANNEX 3. STRESS VULNERABILITY SCALE

(Adapted from Le. H. Miller and Smith's Self-Analysis Model) Name:

Instructions:
In this template you will find 16 topics related to habits and difficulties that most people go through at one time or another. Your frank and honest answers will help us to understand you better.
Rate each item with scores between 1 and 5 according to how often you do each of the following statements, or the degree to which it corresponds to your situation according to the scale below:
1-Always.

2-Most of the time.

3-Frequently.

4-Almost never.

5-Never.

a)   At least four nights a week I sleep seven to eight hours.

b)   Within 50 kilometres I have at least one family I can trust.

c)   At least twice a week I exercise until I sweat.

d)   I smoke less than half a pack of cigarettes a day.

e)   I have less than five drinks (of alcoholic beverages) per week.

f)   I am the right weight for my height.

g)   My income meets my basic expenses

h)   I regularly attend social activities.

i)   I have a network (group) of known friends.

j)   I have one or more friends to whom I can confide my personal problems.

k)   I am in good health (i.e. my eyesight, hearing, teeth are in good condition).

l)   I regularly discuss domestic problems (i.e. housework, money, daily life problems) with the people I live with.

m)   At least once a week I do something for fun.

n)   I am able to organise my time rationally.

o)   I drink at least three cups of coffee, tea or soft drinks a day.

p)   During the day I dedicate some quiet time to myself.

Qualification: It is carried out taking into account:

• Quantitative aspects: The score obtained by the subject will be taken into account; it is clear that the higher the score, the greater the vulnerability to stress. The score that would indicate the lowest level of vulnerability (ideal) would be 16 and the score that would indicate a maximum level of vulnerability would be 80 (theoretically).
To find the quantitative data, add the total of the figures for each question and subtract 16 from the result. The scales are as follows:
☐ Vulnerability to stress: If you accumulate between 24 and 39.

☐ Seriously vulnerable to stress; If it accumulates between 40 and 60

☐ Extremely vulnerable to stress: If the figures exceed 60 points.

ANNEX 4. FAMILY FUNCTIONING PERCEPTION TEST (FF-SIL TEST)
OBJECTIVE: TO ASSESS FAMILY FUNCTIONING.

Below is a group of situations that may or may not occur in your family. You should rank and mark your answer with an X according to how often the situation occurs.

Situations:	Almost never	Rarely	A times	Many times	Almost Always
1 Se taken decisions for things					
important family members.					
2 Harmony prevails in my house. In my house everyone fulfils his or her					
responsibilities					
3 The manifestations of affection					
Form part of our life					
4 daily.We express ourselves without innuendo,					
in a clear and straightforward manner.					
We can accept the shortcomings of the					
5 and cope with them, We take					
in consideration of the experiences of					
Other families to situations					
difficult.					
6 When someone in the family has					
If you have a problem, others help you.					
7 Tasks are distributed as follows					
that no one is overburdened.					
8 Family customs can					
be amended to certain					
situations.					
We can discuss different topics					
9 without fear.					
Faced with a difficult family situation					
10 we are able to seek help in					

	other people.					
	The interests and needs of each					
11	which are respected by the core					
	family.					
12	We show each other the affection we have for each other					
	we have.					

The final score of the test is obtained from the sum of the points per item. The scale has different values according to the selected criterion:

Scale values: *Almost always 5, Many times 4, Sometimes 3, Rarely 2, Almost-neverDiagnosis* ***of Family Functioning according to FF-SIL Test Total Score.***

FUNCTIONAL 70 to 57 point

MODERATELY FUNCTIONAL56 to 43 points

DISFUNCTIONALFrom 42 to 28 points

SEVERELY DYSFUNCTIONALFrom 27 to 14 points

ANNEX SB. FAMILY FUNCTIONING PERCEPTION TEST (FF-SIL) DATA RECORDING MATRIX

SITUATIONS	1. CN		2. PV		3. AV		4. MV		5. CS	
	No	%	No.	%	No.	%	No.	%	No.	%
1										
2										
3										
4										
5										
6										
7										
8										
9										
10										
11										
12										
13										
14										
Total										

Legend: Scenarios 1 to 14 (Annex 5)

ANNEX 6

Table 1. Distribution of diabetic patients according to age and sex. Age Sex Total Female Male

	No.	%	No.	%	No.	%
60 a 64	4	6.78	4	6.78	8	13.56
65 a 69	9	15.25	4	6.78	13	22.03
70 a 74	3	5.08	12	20.34	15	25.42
75 a 79	14	23.73	4	6.78	18	30.51
80 and over.	2	3.39	3	5.08	5	8.47
Total	32	54.24	27	45.76	59	100.00

Source: Individual medical records and questionnaire.

ùTable 2. Distribution of diabetic patients according to sociodemographic variables.

Skin colour

VariablesDiabetic patients	No.	%
Blanca	52	88.13
No White	7	11.86
Out of School	18	30.51
Primary	16	27.12
SchoolingSecondary	5	8.47
Skilled Worker	10	16.95
Pre-university	7	11.86
University.	3	5.08
Housewife	22	37.29
OccupationSelf-employed	20	33.90
State worker	9	15.25
Retired	8	13.56

Source: medical records

Distribution of diabetic patients according to clinical characteristics.

VariablesDiabetic patientsNo. % Diabetic patientsNo. % Diabetic patientsNo. % Diabetic patients

With a background of diabetic relatives **38 64.41**
No record **21 35.59**
Associated comorbidities

Obesity	40	67.80
Primary Hyperlipoproteinaemias	40	67.80
Arterial Hypertension	23	38.98
History of Ischaemic Heart Disease	12	20.34
Chronic kidney disease	3	5.08

Source: medical records

Table 4. Distribution of diabetic patients according to lifestyle determinants and sex.

Sex
Lifestyle determinants

Female n=32 Male n=27Total

		Female n=32		Male n=27		Total	
Stress	32	100,00	27	100,00	59	100,00
Inadequate diet	22	68,75	24	88,89	46	77,97
Sedentary lifestyle	19	59,38	15	55,56	34	57,63
Alcoholism	2	6,25	15	55,56	17	28,81
Light smoker	5	15,63	3	11,11	8	13,56
Moderate smoker	5	15,63	1	3,70	6	10,17
Smoking Severe smoking	21	65,63	22	81,48	43	72,88
Ex-smoker	1	3,13	1	3,70	2	3,39
Subtotal	32	100	27	100	59	100

Source: Individual health history and spinal test*%.

Table 5. Distribution of diabetic patients according to Family Functioning

Family functioning	No.	%
Functional	36	61.02
Moderately functional	16	27.12
Dysfunctional	5	8.47
Severely dysfunctional	2	3.39
Total	59	100.00

Source:FF-SIL Test

Figure 1. Distribution of diabetic patients according to family functioning.

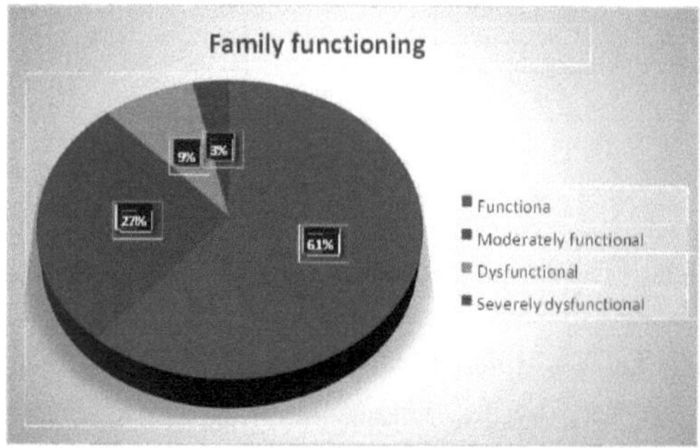

Source: Table 5

Table 6. Distribution of diabetic patients according to lifestyle determinants and glycaemic control. Glycaemic control

Determinantes de estilo de vida	Bien controlados		Descontrol ligero		Descontrol grave	
	No.	%	No.	%	No.	%
Alcoholismo	0	0.00	3	5.08	14	23.72
Sedentarismo	1	1.69	9	15.25	24	40.67
Dieta inadecuada	0	0.00	21	35,59	25	42,37
Estrés	**6**	**10.16**	**28**	**47.45**	**25**	**42.37**
Tabaquismo Fumador leve	8	13,56	0	0.00	0	0.00
Fumador moderado	6	10.16	0	0.00	0	0.00
Fumador severo	0	0.00	28	47.45	25	42,37
Exfumador	2	3.39	0	0.00	0	0.00
Total	**6**	**10.16**	**28**	**47.45**	**25**	**42,37**

Source: Individual health history and spinal test*%.

52

Table 7. Distribution of diabetic patients according to lifestyle determinants and complications.

Complications Foot ulcer Retinopathy Neuropathy Disease Lifestyle determinants of diabetic diabetes Nephropathies diabetic cardiac moderate+

No.	%	No.	%	No.	%	No.	%	No.	%
Alcoholism3	5.08	3	5.08	3	5.08	17	28.81	17	28.81
Sedentary lifestyle10	6.95	3	5.08	0	0.00	15	25.42	34	57,63
Inadequate diet10	16.95	3	5.08	3	5.08	20	33.89	34	57,63
Stress10	16.95	3	5.08	3	5.08	20	33.89	34	57,63
Smoker slightly 0	0.00	0	0.00	0	0.00	0	0.00	1	1.69
Smoker 3	5.08	0	0.00	0	0.00	1	1.69	3	5.08
Tabaquis Smoker 5 Mo severo	8.47	3	5.08	3	5.08	19	32,20	28	47.45
Ex-smoker2	3.39	0	0.00	0	0.00	9	15.25	2	3.39
Total10	16.95	3	5.08	3	5.08	20	33.90	34	57.63

Source: Individual health history and spinal test*%.

Table 8. Distribution of diabetic patients according to economic status and glycaemic control

Glycaemic control Economic situation

Well controlled Out of control light Serious lack of control Total

	No.	%	No.	%	No.	%	No.	%
High:	4	6.78	17	28.81	5	8.47	26	44,06
Medium High:	1	1.69	0	0.00	8	13.56	9	15.25
Average: between	0	0.00	9	15.25	2	3.39	11	18.64
Medium Low:	0	0.00	2	3.39	6	10.16	8	13,56
Low:	1	1.69	0	0.00	4	6.78	5	8.47
Total	6	10.16	28	47.45	25	42,37	59	100.00

Source: Individual health history and spinal test*%.

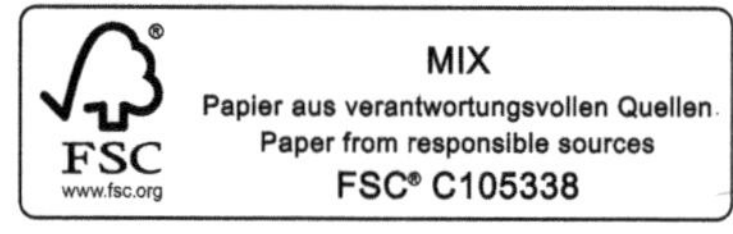

Printed by Books on Demand GmbH, Norderstedt / Germany